CONTENTS

FOREWORD

Those of you who know Roy Lilley will be aware of the problems and pleasures of working with him. If you can imagine travelling at 150 miles an hour in a *Ferrari*, without a seat belt, through a tight chicane, knitting a cardigan, whilst Roy discusses the latest facts he has discovered and asks your opinion on everything from web sites to politics, then you understand.

When we first discussed the possibility of a book on risk management, I admit that I under-estimated Roy's immense enthusiasm. It was no time at all before he agreed to write it and very little more time before I was deluged with instructions requesting information about the chapter headings and the collection of material. Roy's insatiable literary appetite gobbled it all up and, in short order, produced the superb book which you now own.

Risk management is not a fad or some sort of gimmick. It is an essential component of modern professional function. It has been vital, though largely unrecognised, for some years and it continues its rise to a position of pre-eminence amongst the non-clinical functions of every clinician in every general practice.

Risk management cannot be ignored. Like life, it is not something anyone can resign from. It is a simple concept. It is the recognition of those areas where dangers lurk in wait, ready to trap the unwary. It is devising the systems which will minimise or eliminate the chances of the risk rearing up and biting. It is an intensely simple concept, often equally intensely difficult to deliver.

This book will tell you how to do it. In a pleasant and non-threatening meander through the complexities of modern general medical practice and the convolutions of regulation it considers issues around clinical activity, finance, communication and IT. It does not so much seek to instruct as to advise, challenge and question. It points out where the mines are buried and proposes means by which it is possible to avoid being blown up.

The threats to general practice will only get worse. More technology means more to go wrong. More education and publicity means more complaints and litigation. More demand means more pressure and less chance for reflection and planning. This is the book without which life will continue to be walked on a tightrope. If just so much as one risk is eliminated it may be that a six figure bill will be avoided.

Use the book to reduce your anxiety levels. All risk is manageable and here is the way to take the strain out of it.

Happy reading

Dr Paul Lambden
St Paul International Insurance Company Ltd
July 1999

MAKING SENSE

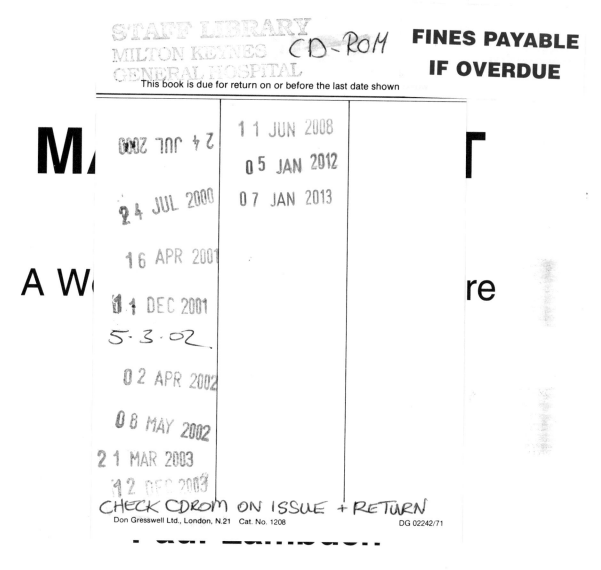

M **T**

A W re

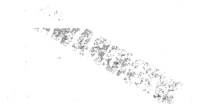

RADCLIFFE MEDICAL PRESS

Radcliffe Medical Press
18 Marcham Road, Abingdon, Oxon OX14 1AA

British Library Cataloguing in Publication Data

A catalogue record for this book is available from the British Library.

ISBN 1 85775 490 5

Typeset in Great Britain
Printed and bound in Great Britain

PREFACE

If the NHS deserves a prize, it must be for having the most baffling jargon of any of our great public services, or for that matter any other administration! The list of buzz phrases, initials and acronyms grows as we speak. Never mind the old faithfuls that have been around for years: DHA, NED, JCC and CHC. In the last few months we have had PCGs, PCTs, NICE and CHImP dumped on us – to name but a few.

The situation is compounded by the fact that although the NHS is not a business, it does recognise that it should try and conduct its affairs in a business like way. Hence, it complicates its already incomprehensible thesaurus with words borrowed from the lexicon of industry.

The NHS is a great one for management fads. I have seen: the vision thing; flat-organisation theory; decoding corporate culture; organisational environment development; empowerment; quality circles; fuzzy logic; the learning organisation; scenario planning; customer focus and reengineering. Each idea is important in its own way, but somehow, often fails to translate into NHS operational management and make the impact that it should.

On the whole I think the NHS is well managed. It is a resource capped, demand led nightmare, that no sane manager would ever dream of getting anywhere near! But, thank goodness, they do. They consistently produce more, for less. By and large the NHS goes about its business in a sensible way and delivers the goods.

My question is: can it last? Recent, spectacular, clinical failures have highlighted the fact that when the NHS gets it wrong, it usually turns out to be a disaster for somebody. The NHS does not make little mistakes. As the NHS's working environment gets more complex and the world becomes increasingly litigious the cost of getting it wrong is a price that becomes increasingly difficult to pay.

Primary care teams, now working in different ways, taking on a greater share of the responsibility for managing their affairs, will come face to face with the dilemmas of managing risks, both clinical and non-clinical, and responding to the uncertainties and problems that all new organisations face.

Can the NHS work in the 'zero-defect' environment of the car, or electronics industry? People aren't Pentium chips and casualties aren't cars on a production line. Clinical protocols and treatment guidelines may remove some of the uncertainties from the equation although they may create as many problems as they resolve. Prescribing support and whatever other neat tricks the Gods of Whitehall might dream up may move us closer to conveyor belt medicine, but the infinite variety and complexity of what the health service does probably means the NHS will continue to get things wrong.

I'm prepared to say there is no great sin in getting something wrong. The sins are: not knowing the organisation is getting something wrong; not knowing how often it gets something wrong; and having no idea how to learn from mistakes and making the commitment that they must never happen again.

To complicate the life of the under-resourced and overwhelmed GP even further, there is another new, neat little phrase, to emerge from the Department of Health. *Clinical Governance*. Clinical governance is a strategy for improving the overall quality of clinical care. It also places a legal duty on some of the key players to get it right – or go to jail. This is starting to get hairy! If you're wondering about clinical governance, there is a great book on the topic, published by Radcliffe (the publishers of this book) but modesty prevents me from identifying the author! *(There's a first for everything – Ed)*. There's also a supplement towards the back of this book, that will give you an idea of what it all means.

Does the language and repertoire of business technique have anything to offer a beleaguered NHS looking to make stepping stones of its mistakes – rather than mill-stones? Well, risk management, a management technique developed in industry as an off shoot of various quality initiatives, is a good place to start. Risk management recognises that all organisations and most activities have risks attached to them. Indeed, the complete avoidance of all risk means never doing anything.

Everything we do, from crossing the road to eating a bag of chips, has a risk. Diagnosing that a child has the 'flu' is a risk; they might have meningitis. Mopping a floor has a risk; someone might slip on a wet bit. Working out a budget has a risk; it might not be right and you could run out of cash.

The principles of risk management are simple enough – figure out what might go wrong and plan for it. Really it's an up market version of Murphy's Law. Murphy's Law says, if something can go wrong it will. The 'up market' bit is about trying to spot it coming and doing something about it, in advance. This workbook falls into the category of 'doing something about it'. It is not about planning for disaster, it is about planning for success. It is about having a methodical, calm look at the organisation and arranging things in such a way as to minimise the chances you are taking, the gambles you are making and removing the uncertainty from what you do. No rocket science, just common sense.

Risk management: one new phrase in the healthcare dictionary that could make a difference to you, where you work and the people you provide a service for.

You could decide to stay in bed. . . Or make sense of risk management with the help of this book. Your call!

Roy Lilley

ABOUT THE AUTHORS

Roy Lilley is a visiting fellow at the Management School, Imperial College London. He is a writer and broadcaster on health and social issues and has published nearly a dozen books on health and health service management and related topics.

As a former NHS Trust chairman his Trust became the first to achieve BS 5750 (ISO 9001), quality accreditation for the whole of their services along with Investors in People approval for the whole of their HR and training strategies.

Roy Lilley now works across the NHS to help with the challenges of modern management and is an enthusiast for radical policies that address the real needs of patients, professionals and the communities they serve.

Paul Lambden is a doctor and a dentist, a former GP and NHS Trust Chief Executive, as well as being a regular writer on medical, health and management topics. For three years he was an adviser to the Health Select Committee and is now the Medical and Dental Principal at St Paul International Insurance Company Ltd.

ACKNOWLEDGEMENTS

Anne O'Connor BSc RM RSCN RN

Ashley Winters

Allan Prangley RGN

Ian Warren BSc, RGN, RMN, Dip N (Lond), MBIM

Bruce Balck RN, BSN, ARM

Dr John Navein MBCHB, MRCGP, DCH, DTM&H, LRCP, MRCS

DEDICATION

All the books in my PCG series have been dedicated to the army of NHS managers, clinicians and medical staff who have influenced my understanding of our greatest public service. I thanked them for the time they had taken and for sharing their insights, knowledge and experiences. I do so again.

It would also be right to thank the professionals in the risk management industry and in particular those at St Paul Insurance who have, patiently, taken me through the issues.

And, once again to A-T R, who takes the biggest risk of all, in trying to manage me!

risk /risk/n & v. – n a chance or possibility of danger, loss, injury, or other adverse consequence

management /mænidjment/ n. the professional administration of business concerns

risk management / risk mænidjment/ incomprehensible guru speak and a task that is somebody else's job

We could try something more sensible:

Risk Management
An insurance and quality control related discipline comprising activities designed to minimise the adverse effects of loss upon a healthcare organisation's human, physical and financial assets, through:

- Identification of loss potential

- Loss prevention and reduction

- Loss funding and Risk Financing

- Claims control

. . . . . . Yup, definitely more sensible but not as much fun as the one over the page!

MAKING THIS BOOK WORK FOR YOU

I'll start by taking a risk! I'll bet you are not the type of person who has the time to sit down and read a book from cover to cover.

See, I knew I was right! Good start, eh?

This book removes the risk of not being read by a non *cover to cover* person – like you. The book has no conventional beginning, middle or end. So, don't feel obliged to sit down and read it from cover to cover in a nice ordered way, because you can't. I don't want you to.

Instead, flip through the pages and get a feel for what it has to offer. Not all of it will be of interest to you – skip those bits. Pick out the sections that look like they can help. This is a workbook so make it <u>work</u> for you. Flip through the pages – make friends with it! Do it now and then come back to this page. By the way, because I am a lazy typist, I've substituted RM for the words *risk management* throughout. . . Make a coffee and have a flip around.

Welcome back!

I hope you have come across things in the book that you know already and hopefully, some things you've never thought of. Perhaps even some stuff to make you think.

A game of two halves

You will have noticed the book is in two parts – the first part explains the mechanics of risk management, the basics of the techniques you will need to 'risk manage' any situation plus a few examples. The second part deals with some specific issues and takes you through the steps you might want to consider in risk managing them.

Also . . .

THINK BOX

There are a number of 'THINK BOXES': they are there to get *the juices flowing* and to get you thinking *outside the box* – look at the issues from a different dimension. Some are deliberately provocative, some just for fun.

 Hazard Warnings are there to point out some tricky issues, or traps not to fall into.

 The Tips are short cuts and quick fixes to get you to the answer faster.

The Exercises are here for you to address the issues in the context of where you work and what your task is – regardless of your profession or seniority in the organisation. Use them to develop your own thinking or for brainstorming the issues with colleagues.

There are a lot of questions and no answers. This is not a 'right' or 'wrong' book; this book asks the questions in the context of the issues in the hope that they will help you not to overlook an important topic or duck some of the tricky ones.

This is a non-threatening, environmentally friendly, non-genetically modified, unashamedly irreverently written, fun to play with book that tries to make RM easy.

Write on the pages, rip bits out, argue with it and throw it at a picture of Frank Dobson (*just an expression – no letters from Millbank Towers, please – Ed*). Use it as a workbook to prove that not everything in life has to be serious to be good. Well, that's the idea – what do you think?

Where do you work?

Here are three *error philosophies* – more guru speak for attitudes towards foul-ups. Which one do you recognise?

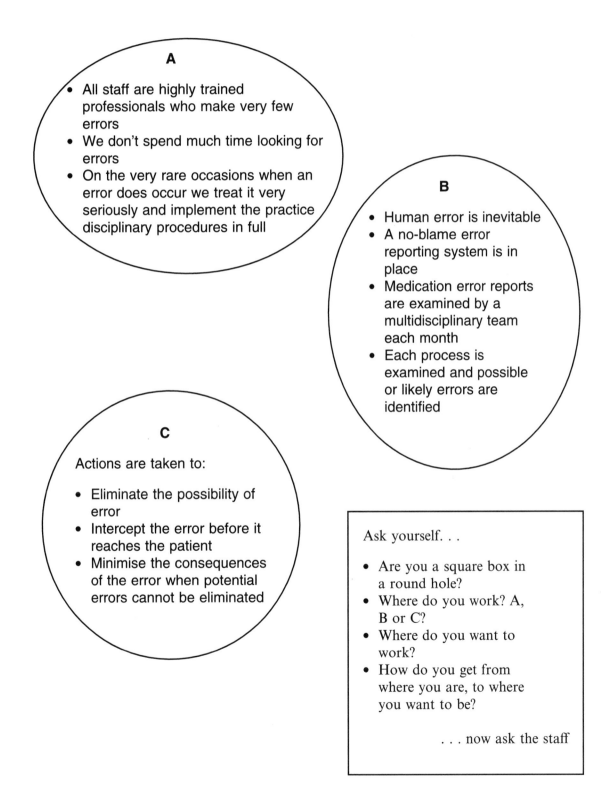

A
- All staff are highly trained professionals who make very few errors
- We don't spend much time looking for errors
- On the very rare occasions when an error does occur we treat it very seriously and implement the practice disciplinary procedures in full

B
- Human error is inevitable
- A no-blame error reporting system is in place
- Medication error reports are examined by a multidisciplinary team each month
- Each process is examined and possible or likely errors are identified

C

Actions are taken to:

- Eliminate the possibility of error
- Intercept the error before it reaches the patient
- Minimise the consequences of the error when potential errors cannot be eliminated

Ask yourself. . .

- Are you a square box in a round hole?
- Where do you work? A, B or C?
- Where do you want to work?
- How do you get from where you are, to where you want to be?

. . . now ask the staff

SECTION 1

Risk, what risk?

Don't know about risk management *(that's the last time I type risk management – from now on it's RM)*, don't worry you're not alone. Here's all you need to know. Just four things. Rip this bit out and stick it, nonchalantly, on the notice board in the office.

Make like you know something!

The Four Principles of Risk Management

1   Identify the risk – *figure out what's likely to foul up.*

2   Analyse the risk – *think about what the chances are of it going wrong, its impact and does it matter.*

3   Control the risk – *is there anything you can do about it?*

4   Cost the risk – *what's the cost of getting it right versus the cost of getting it wrong?*

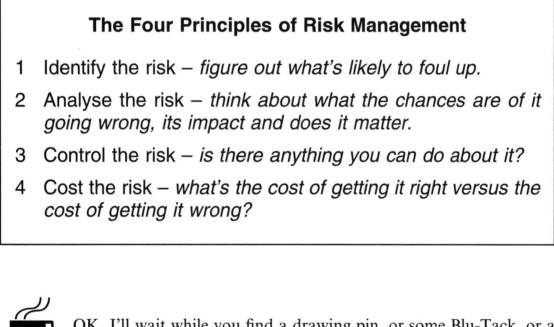 OK, I'll wait while you find a drawing pin, or some Blu-Tack, or a nail, or tape, or something – please try and be a bit more organised, will you!

So, what's the difference between:

- Clinical risk management
- Financial risk management
- . . . and risk management?

Answer: Nothing

The answer is printed upside down to annoy the printer and to try and give you some exercise whilst you read the book.

The fact is, risk management is risk management. Whether you run a chip shop or an operating theatre. Whether you are in tree surgery or in your surgery, the principles are the same. What are the principles? Look at your notice board and remind yourself. Or, if you haven't got round to ripping the page out of the book and to save you the sweat of having to turn the page, here they are again:

The Four Principles of Risk Management

1 Identify the risk – *figure out what's likely to foul up.*

2 Analyse the risk – *think about what the chances are of it going wrong, its impact and does it matter.*

3 Control the risk – *is there anything you can do about it?*

4 Cost the risk – *what's the cost of getting it right versus the cost of getting it wrong?*

  OK, I'll wait while you find a drawing pin, or some Blu-Tack. *(Please!)*

What does it all mean?

Isn't this just another exercise in bureaucracy?

Do you want an honest answer? OK, the answer is, yes. Well, maybe. Er, probably. Mmm, perhaps. And, I know you are busy and I know you don't have any spare time and if you did you'd spend it on something interesting like your collection of fine wines or making friends with the strange people who share your house – called the family.

BUT – yes it is a big **BUT**, just stop and think for a moment. How much of your time do you already take up with things like:

- Audit

- Claims

- Complaints

- Planning & review

- Adverse incident reporting

- Education & training

. . . the answer is, if you're honest – a long time.

The whole idea of RM *(remember, from now on RM stands for risk management)*, is to get better organised and avoid the necessity of spending time fixing things up after they've gone wrong. Investing some time, up front, will pay dividends in the longer run and improve the quality of care your team provides. So let's stop paper exercises and do something positive with the information.

What sort of issues does RM cover?

THE 3 AIMS OF CLINICAL RISK MANAGEMENT

- Reducing or eliminating harm to the patient.

- Dealing with the injured patient and supporting clinical staff.

- Safeguarding the assets of the organisation.

Here's the philosophical point: just like in the real world outside the surgery (*yes, there is one*), there are risks in everything we do. Here are some of the areas of risk in an average practice:

- Not being up to date with the best clinical practice or the latest technical and pharmaceutical development

- Getting something wrong, for a patient

- A break down in the continuity of care for the patient, across the interfaces with other bodies and services

- Breakdown in communication

- Patient complaints

- Failing to safeguard the assets of the practice – the building and the bits and pieces in it

- Financial risks – running out of cash

- Risks to reputation – yours and your colleagues

- Risks to staff morale – making sure they don't get the hump and leave.

So whose job is it?

Everyone has a part to play in RM, just like they do with clinical governance. However, common sense tells us, someone senior should take a lead. As you can see the risks are diverse, clinical, managerial and goodness knows what else.

So, here's the first exercise.

Exercise

Under the arrangements for clinical governance, the PCG must appoint a responsible person for delivering the quality agenda. Is it a good idea for the lead on clinical governance to be the lead on RM? Is it desirable or practical to combine the roles? Consider the whole breadth of risk. Think about the advantages and disadvantages of sharing the task and joint roles. What are the likely areas of conflict? At a practice level, is it practical to divide the responsibilities? Could the various practices that make up a PCG provide an element of RM each contributing to the big picture? Would this provide an 'interface problem'?

An 'interface' is the point at which one group hands over to the next; there is the potential to drop the baton, a point at which no one is responsible. Think of it as a set of paving stones. The point at which the smooth surfaces meet, the join, is the bit that people trip over; break the neck of their femur and you know the rest!

So, how do we go about it?

We gotta have a system

Good management is simple enough. There are loadsa management gurus who will take loadsa money off you, in the name of getting you sorted out and maybe, in time, you might need some help. But, before you start splashing the taxpayers pounds around, here are the basics.

Nobody tells me anything, I just work here!

I bet you've heard that before! It's the mushroom syndrome. Keep people in the dark, throw enough manure at them and expect them to grow. It might work for the Agricus Arvensis *(Horse Mushroom, to you)*, but not for a district nurse or health visitor or a receptionist or the senior partner.

RM is an inclusive approach and an attempt to run a more efficient and safe organisation. It is <u>inclusive</u>. Efficient and safe places are good places to work. No one wants to be at risk or to work in a muddle.

Think of RM as the stripe in a tube of toothpaste. It goes right through. So, staff working in the practice cannot be expected to participate, properly, unless they know what is going on and what they are supposed to contribute.

You gotta tell 'em.

Exercise

 Design an approach to inform staff what RM is, what the benefits to them might be and how they can play their part.

Look at the exercise, first from the practice point of view and then imagine your practice is taking the lead on communicating a RM initiative across a whole PCG. Against that background what techniques would you use to communicate across the whole range of professionals that are likely to be involved?

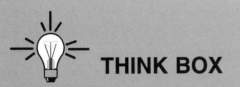 **THINK BOX**

PCGs are encouraged to develop better working relationships outside health. Social Services, housing authorities and the voluntary sector are all involved in modern healthcare planning and service delivery. Should these professionals be involved in your RM initiatives? Is it reasonable to expect them to participate and to subscribe to your methods of working and quality standards?

What's so risky?

Maybe this is not such a tough question. Most people know where the risks are. You don't have to work somewhere, for too long, to figure out who the dodgy practitioners and systems are... But, it doesn't have to be as tricky as that. Risks are risks, wherever they are. The edge of that carpet, that is curling up in the doorway to the waiting room. That's risk. Someone could trip. Whose job is it to tape it down, nail it, rip it up or buy a new carpet?

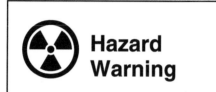

Hazard Warning

You can criticise a doctor's driving, you can criticise their golf swing. You might even get away with criticising their performance between the sheets, but you'd better not have a go at their clinical practice!

What about the extension socket that is powering three PCs, the photocopier and the electric kettle!

At this point I can hear you saying, this is very basic stuff, Roy! You're right. Whoever said management was difficult? Identifying risks doesn't have to be difficult. The difficulty seems to be doing something about them.

Let's look at some trickier areas.

Have you, your colleagues, or the docs you work with, ever had to make a claim, or seek the advice of their medical negligence insurers? Oh, now that is difficult! Folk get very touchy about that sort of question.

You can criticise a doctor's driving, you can criticise their golf swing. You might even get away with criticising their performance between the sheets, but you'd better not have a go at their clinical practice!

Handling criticism isn't easy. Do it sensitively.

However, a doctor's claims history is a good indicator of where risks might be.

Exercise

How would you approach gathering information about a doctor's medical negligence claims history? What special steps might you have to consider to keep information confidential and preserve the dignity of the medic?

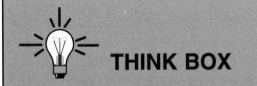

THINK BOX

Should claims made by a doctor, against his professional indemnity insurance be a matter of public record? Is the public entitled to know about a doctor's performance?

Starting to get the picture?

What about other areas of clinical risk?

Not being up to date with the latest clinical practice might lead to unnecessary risks being taken with patient care. Practices get deluged with information from pharmaceutical companies, the medical press and the Department of Health. In an effort to keep up to date, if every doc read everything that was put in front of them, they would probably never have time to see patients!

Exercise

    Devise a system to ensure the GPs in your practice are kept up to date with the latest developments in clinical practice. What sources of information would you use and how could you be sure it was reliable?

Phew, that was close!

British Airways have a neat system for reporting what they call 'near misses'. They accept, from time to time, something might go wrong. It doesn't have to be a disaster, it can be quite a little thing. They understand that to avoid disasters they must pay attention to the little things, in a way that encourages staff to report a near miss, in a 'no-blame' environment. British Airways want to learn about why things go wrong and they can't do that unless they know what is going wrong.

Exercise

Consider the potential for near miss episodes in your practice. How would you collect information on near misses? What reporting systems could you devise, formal or informal, to capture information about things that very nearly went wrong? What tools would you use to analyse the data and how would you disseminate it so that others could learn from the experience?

Blowing the whistle?

Finding out where the real risks are is sometimes next to impossible unless someone is prepared to *blow the whistle*. To help manage this a well designed and supported accident/incident reporting system is essential. This will identify both failures in the system and in individual practice. The accident and incident reporting system will not work unless staff feel that confidentiality is assured and that those individuals identified as having serious or frequent incidents are supported or retrained as necessary. Disciplinary measures are taken only as a last resort.

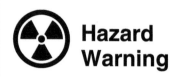

Hazard Warning

If someone wants to blow the whistle how easy is it for your organisation to hear it?

How do you separate out the meddlesome from the well intended?

Exercise

Devise arrangements for concerns to be reported. What assurances would you put into the system to ensure confidentiality and to sort genuine concerns from the mendacious?

THINK BOX

Whistle blowing, now there's a mistake to start with. How did we end up with a phrase like whistle blowing?

Do you want to be branded a *whistle blower*? No! I bet you don't and I don't think anyone in their right mind would want that epithet to stick. Whistle blowing, a phrase that was dumped on the NHS by the tabloids and management journals, has stuck. Not only has it stuck, it has also been adopted by the NHS, as a short hand title for a range of very difficult issues indeed. It may be short hand but it is also very short sighted. Sends out all the wrong kind of messages!

There must be a fair few folk who might be tempted to express their concerns about the clinical practice, or conduct of a colleague, in confidence. But not if they are going to end up branded a *whistle blower*. Let's start a campaign to eradicate the words from the NHS dictionary.

Exercise

Brainstorm with colleagues and find a new phrase for wh~~is~~. . . you know what. If you find a good one – let me know!

Somebody out there is saying something about you!

Did you know that research in service industries indicates that the total number of people who complain often represents less than 6% of the total of those who might have just cause to complain, they just can't be bothered! So, if that data holds good for the NHS, take the number of complaints you had last year and figure out what another 94% might do to the totals. Ugh, doesn't bear thinking about, does it?

The British are not great complainers. They are getting better at it. The number of complaints the NHS deals with is going up. What do we do with complaints once we've sorted them?

In industry, customer complaints are taken very seriously. They are used as a tool to redesign systems and products and to benchmark and measure progress. I'm not so sure about the NHS. The Health Service seems to regard complaints as an unjustifiable intrusion into the working day!

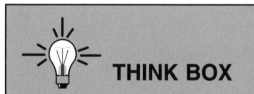 **THINK BOX**

Three out of four people who sue the NHS do so for reasons other than money:

• One in five said they wanted information and the court room was the only place they could get it

• One in five said they thought the doctors were hiding something

• One in three subsequent treating doctors implied, or declared, that the original care was substandard.

Complaints can be a very good way of measuring and forecasting risk. If complaints about similar things keep popping up – there's a risk.

If different people find a problem with the same thing, the chances are it's not the people who are the problem.

Evidence from insurance companies suggests that claims against doctors are not random. Docs at risk of being complained against are described by their patients as:

- Rushing them
- Ignoring them
- Giving them too little information.

Does that sound like anyone at your surgery!

The ones least likely to be complained about:

- Laughed and used humour
- Used 'orientation statements' (that's guru speak for phrases such as '*what do you expect now?*' and '*in the future*')
- Sought the patient's opinion: '*what do you think the problem is?*'
- Had consultations that built relationships: '*what concerns do you have?*' or '*Tell me more*'
- Were active listeners: '*what do you think caused the problem?*'

Recognise anyone?

Docs ain't saints

In the real world we know, we get rushed and feel overworked, under appreciated and underpaid! It is easy to forget that a doc offers more than a diagnosis, people have feelings and they are sensitive, often vulnerable in the surgery. In a busy surgery it is easy to get into *conveyor belt* mode. Conscious of the patients piling up in the waiting room the temptation is to 'move people through the system'.

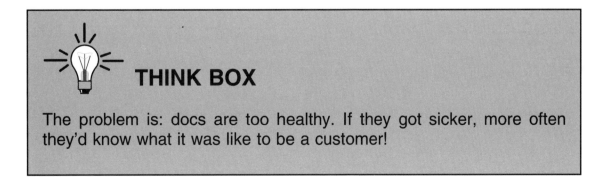

THINK BOX

The problem is: docs are too healthy. If they got sicker, more often they'd know what it was like to be a customer!

Exercise

Evaluate your practice's complaints procedures and devise a way of using complaints as a risk management tool, spotting trends and identifying 'hot spots'. Could your system be rolled out across more than one practice? Can it be used, or adapted as a RM tool for the whole PCG?

The current NHS complaints procedures were put in place in 1996. The aim was to:

- Make it easier for people to complain

- Make the complaints procedure simpler

- Separate out complaints from the disciplinary procedures

- Make the process fairer

- Resolve problems and satisfy the concerns of the complainant.

That was three years ago – what's happened since? Complaints have gone up, that's true but the number of disciplinary proceedings against GPs has gone down, dramatically.

When is a complaint not a complaint? Good question. A patient may complain about anything: relatively minor or something very serious. Whatever the cause of the complaint, it is important to the person complaining. In the words of the American business management guru, Tom Peters, *'perception is everything'*.

Two things can be guaranteed to make a complaint worse: not getting a fair hearing and not receiving a full explanation of the facts of the case.

A complaint may be in writing, oral, or received through a third party. The process of resolving complaints has several potential stages: local resolution, lay conciliation, independent review, and Ombudsman review.

Here's how the process works:

Local resolution

The aim, here, is twofold:

- Investigate, resolve and/or take action

- To respond to the complainant as quickly as possible as close to the initial complaint as possible.

Some practices appoint a manager responsible for complaints. Their job is to:

- maintain timetables

- organise responses

- advise complainants on their rights

- monitor process and time scales

- protect patient rights.

. . . and most important of all, find a resolution which satisfies everyone involved.

The best way to resolve a complaint, locally, is to try to have a face to face meeting (docs are good at that sort of thing). Be sure to keep a full note of the meeting and, if possible, have it in the presence of a third party. In any case, best practice is to respond fully in writing.

Be sure to keep the complainant informed and advise them where to get help – the CHC or Citizen's Advice Bureau are good places to start.

Very important: <u>be sure to keep notes</u> on meetings with a complainant. Don't get upset, however rotten the experience and avoid antagonism at all costs.

New kid on the block

Enter a new character – stage left. . .

There is a new player in the complaints drama, employed by the health authority – the *lay conciliator*. He or she is available to both the doctor and the patient. Their job is to find a way through the difficulties. The conciliator reviews correspondence, speaks to the complainant and doctor, investigates, seeks appropriate independent advice and writes a full informative letter to both parties.

The complainant then has 28 days to decide whether to request an Independent Review. This is considered by the Convenor. The Convenor is a lay member of the HA. Don't worry, they take advice on clinical issues.

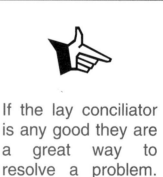

If the lay conciliator is any good they are a great way to resolve a problem. Ask around, see what colleagues' experiences have been.

The Convenor decides:

- Whether an Independent Review would *ADD VALUE* to the resolution. (Strange phrase, but it is in the Guidance on the topic. Does sort of sum up the bother or not to bother question though, don't ya think?)

- Discusses the issues with the putative Chair of the Review.

If the decision is that a Review would be helpful, the Convenor makes sure the terms of reference are reasonable.

The lay chair is nominated by the Regional Office of the NHS Management executive on behalf of the Secretary of State *(big stuff this)*.

Once an Independent Review (IR) is agreed, the Chair takes control of the process and works within the terms of reference. Who does the paper work and writes and circulates draft and final reports?

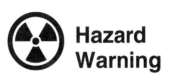

Hazard Warning

Doctors should take an Independent Review very seriously. Although it is not linked with disciplinary proceedings, if a doctor is censured in an Independent Review the Chief Executive of the Health Authority can decide to institute proceedings. Docs are advised to prepare well, establishing clear explanations and arguments. Although the GP cannot take a lawyer to a review meeting, they should be accompanied by a defence body adviser or LMC secretary. Do not go alone – even if you do fancy yourself as Perry Mason.

How does it work?

An IR panel consists of:

1 Chairman (appointed by Regional Office on behalf of the Secretary of State)

2 Convenor (who is a lay member of the HA)

3 Third Panel member (independent person nominated by the Secretary of State)

4 Two independent medical advisers, usually nominated by the professional body, the LMC.

The complainant and doctor can be seen either separately or together. Each is questioned by members of the panel. Either may make a statement.

The idea is for the Chairman to satisfy the doctor and the complainant *(sounds like a job for Solomon) (Well, certainly not for you – Ed)* and to produce recommendations which could produce improvements in service quality, efficiency and effectiveness.

After IR and within 30 working days of the appointment of the panel *(so this is a process that gets on with the job – no hanging about)* the Chairman must produce a draft report and send a copy to the complainant and doctor for comment. The final report is sent to the Chief Executive of the Health Authority, to the complainant and the doctor.

This is the important bit. It is the Chief Executive's job to decide whether to take disciplinary action against a GP. If so, a service hearing is convened. This is rare and would be rarer still if docs took the process as seriously as they should.

The Ombudsman (Health Service Commissioner) can be approached by either complainant or doctor and may investigate: if there is injustice or hardship on either the doctor or the patient; if decisions fell out-of-time; or if there was a decision to refuse an Independent Review which the patient feels is unfair.

The Ombudsman investigates less than 5% of cases referred to him though he may write to the parties expressing a view about an application. He will not investigate complaints that are still on-going and will not investigate disciplinary matters.

There are five key objectives in the complaints process:

1 Try to find agreement between complainant and doctor

2 Obtain written evidence where possible

3 Support evidence with independent witnesses

4 Identify issues in the report

5 Separate fact from disputed events.

How long does it all take?

A complaint must be made within 6 months of the event
OR
within 6 months of becoming aware of the cause for complaint
AND
no longer than 12 months from event (there is some discretion to extend the timescale).

Local resolution timetable

Oral complaints can be dealt with on the spot or referred to the complaints procedures.
Written complaints must be acknowledged in 3 working days
OR
if no acknowledgement is provided a full reply must be sent in 5 working days.

If the complaint is acknowledged, then a full reply must be sent within 10 working days.

After the response (and conciliation if taken up) the complainant has a further 28 calendar days to seek an IR.

Next

- IR Convenor must acknowledge a request for a Review in 2 working days

- The decision to establish a panel must be made within 10 working days of receipt of request

- The appointment of the panel must be made in a further 10 working days

- Draft report must be produced within 30 working days of formal appointment of panel

- The final report produced within a further 10 working days

- Report circulated within 5 further working days.

Note the switch at the *response from complainant* stage, from working days to calendar days.

If you'd like to save yourself all this grief, here are 10 ways to reduce risk in handling complaints.

Ten tips for handling complaints

1 Take every complaint seriously

2 Talk to people – you are good at it!

3 Do not write aggressive replies

4 Apologise for any mistakes

5 It is not just the patient who sees your responses. Ensure your replies will sound reasonable to a Convenor, CHC or lawyer

6 If conciliation is suggested, go for it. In any decisions about, or by, an IR, refusing conciliation may weigh against you

7 Do not go to an IR alone – take a friend/defence organisation/LMC representative

8 A spoonful of sugar is good in IRs. Do not lose your temper with the panel, even if they do deserve it!

9 Ensure written evidence for the panel is ordered, neat and easy to digest – particularly for the lay members

10 Supporting witnesses can be very valuable.

What if it all goes pear shaped and you end up with a claim against you?

Complaints are a key area of risk for a doctor. They can be seriously career threatening. However, careful management of complaints can often lead to the resolution of the problem without the need to resort to hearings and what have you. Also, well managed complaints often don't develop into anything nasty.

It is often the second insult that brings on the red mist and the patient reaches for the complaint button. It is often not the initial event that causes the patient to complain. It is the fact that their complaint is badly handled or they are otherwise fobbed off.

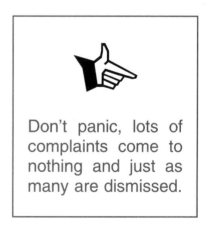

Don't panic, lots of complaints come to nothing and just as many are dismissed.

We are witnessing the *customerisation* of healthcare. Gone are the days of deference to doctors. Patients 'know their rights'.

Whether a patient is buying a tin of sardines in the supermarket or having his bunions sorted out in the surgery – they want to be treated like a customer.

The new disciplinary procedures are:

- Easy for patients to access
- Simple to understand
- Designed to separate complaints from disciplinary procedures
- Aimed at encouraging everyone involved to 'learn the lessons from complaints'
- Fairer to staff and complainants
- Faster and get the complaint dealt with quickly.

The Complainant:
- Has the right to be heard
- To be taken seriously
- To request independent review
- To refer complaint to Ombudsman, CHC and GMC.

And, has the responsibility to:
- Provide a statement of outstanding issues
- Explain why they are still dissatisfied
- Respond within time scales
- Respect the process.

By the way the complainant does not have a <u>right</u> to:
- An independent review
- Violate staff rights
- Have non-NHS work investigated under NHS procedures
- Restart the process if they are still dissatisfied
- Demand any particular action or result.

Knock, knock – who's there? A postman with a letter of claim against you!

If you receive a letter of claim it will usually be in the form of a solicitor's letter. Do not panic. Solicitors are unpleasant people who write threatening letters – they can't help it. It's something in their genes. Send the letter straight to your defence organisation. Let them worry about it – that's what you pay them for!

Under the new reforms proposed by Lord Justice Woolf the process must be done *speedily*. (Nice turn of phrase these legal bods have, don't you think?)

Whadaya gonna do?

Claims may be settled or defended. Discuss the options with your defence organisation. Make sure the discussions are detailed and they keep you fully informed of developments as they unfold. If you are kept in the dark, change your insurer.

THINK BOX

There may be a range of factors that govern whether you defend or settle. Which is best for you? Only you will know. For example, it will be of no value to go to court and win, if the local press vilifies you and destroys your practice. A hollow victory indeed. And, then you'll have another battle on your hands with the Press Complaints Council.

Ten tips for dealing with claims

1 Do nothing without the agreement of your defence organisation

2 Send all correspondence straight to them and get on with your life

3 Collect together any evidence which might be of value

4 Do not deface, destroy or otherwise alter any notes, letters or other material *(That sounds official don't it? – Ed)*

5 Tell the truth to your defence organisation. Don't embellish, tell a little porky or duck a difficult bit. Tell the stripped-pine, God's honest – however embarrassing. There's nothing you can do that they haven't come across before. Telling them what the bottom line is gives you and them the best chance of the least damaging settlement

6 Do not let anger cloud your judgement about the most pragmatic solution. Bung your pride in your back pocket, get a grip and get on with your life

7 Witnesses are valuable – have you got any, can you get any?

8 Because of the changes in the procedures, timescales are very tight. Do not delay – if someone wants information provide it, pronto!

9 Remember that experts may not agree with your assessment of the management of the case. If your defence adviser tells you that experts are united in disagreeing with your approach, put your explanation for your actions carefully but remember that the test in the UK at least is still what a *reasonable* body of practitioners would do. So try and be reasonable!

10 Try not to start from here! Watch out for the potential claim and nip it in the bud. The medical protection folk tell me that most cases could have been avoided for the sake of a little thought earlier on.

Changes in the way the legal profession is organised and remunerated are likely to mean more 'no win, no fee' cases. Lawyers have got to earn a living, just like everyone else. Never get angry with a lawyer – get even – win your case!

Exercise

Audit the complaints received by your practice over the last 24 months against requirements for the timeliness of the responses. What percentage of complaints are dealt with within the required time limits? What processes can you put in place to ensure a higher level of compliance?

Is it possible to avoid complaints?

Probably not all of them. However, there are some RM tricks that can reduce the likelihood of complaints. They are called *tone setting* – that's guru speak for creating an atmosphere that appears open and accessible, where comments are welcomed and acted upon and no one makes a drama out of a complaint. Where can you see it in action? Try Marks and Sparks – they've got it down to a fine art.

How can you do it? Easy:

Foster an environment that allows patients to provide feedback.

Use:
- Survey forms
- Have a 'hot-line' or patient relations person who can deal with an issue promptly
- Ensure complaints are dealt with extra-super-whizzo fast responses

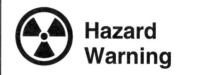

Hazard Warning

Survey after survey, in health and outside, shows that people who complain want four things:

- To be taken seriously
- Clear up the problem so it can never happen again
- Immediate action
- To be listened to.

- Train staff to understand why people complain and not to feel threatened by complaints.

When survey data has been gathered – publish the results, even if it is bad news. And then, here's the important bit, publish what you intend to do about it. Give some time for the changes to take effect, re-survey and publish the results and measure the improvements.

The do's and don't of reducing the risk of complaints

- Don't be defensive
- Do say: 'Oh dear, I am sorry to hear you have cause to complain, please tell me about it'
- Don't cite policy and say 'It's the system'.
- Do say: 'It doesn't matter what the procedures are, we need to try and get this right for you'
- Do listen, do take notes and do ask questions

- Don't pass the buck: 'I'm sorry you're not my patient'
- Do say: 'I'm sorry to hear this. I may not be the best person to help you but tell me what's happened and I'll see how I can help'.

Keep a proper record of the complaint

Write down:

- The patient's name
- How to contact them
- Background information on the situation, time, people involved, what happened
- How the patient defined the problem
- What you agreed to do
- Suggestion you have regarding the solution
- Action and follow up.

Avoiding complaints is not just about *doing the right thing*, it's about setting the right atmosphere.

Do you:

- Always keep the patient informed, such things as the examination process and why
- Leave the room when the patient is changing
- Knock before re-entering the room
- Respect cultural differences such as age, race, religion or ethnicity

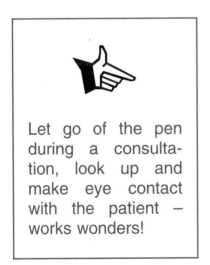

Let go of the pen during a consultation, look up and make eye contact with the patient – works wonders!

No, no's

What upsets patients? Here are a few headliners from a patient survey!

- Inappropriate touching – such as putting an arm around a patient's waist
- Kissing a patient hello or goodbye
- Asking about marital status (out of context)
- Holding a hand and not letting go
- Complimenting on looks or attractiveness.

Honest, that's what patients say. You couldn't make it up! Some people just ask for trouble and boy, do they get it!

The cursed phone

The first contact most patients have with the surgery is over the phone. You'd think, by the way some people behave on the phone, it had just been invented. Practice staff who answer the telephone, in some practices, are some of the worst phone users I have ever come across. Mainly it's because they are busy and receive so little training. It is a shame because they set the tone for the whole relationship between the patient and the practice.

Here is a *'one side of a piece of A4'* crammer on handling the phone. Rip this page out and copy it to all the people who answer the phone over at your place. To hell with the copyright laws – I give you my permission!

- When you pick up the phone – smile. I promise you, you can hear a smile over the phone.
- Never make an important phone call sitting down. You can hear body language over the phone, too. Honest!
- Answer with the name of the organisation and your name – forget the 'how may I help you' rubbish. When you say the name of the practice, say it slowly, like it was the first time. You may have said it 50 times in the morning but it will be the first time the caller has heard it.
- Address the caller by their proper name: Mrs Brown, not madam or dear.
- If you have to put the caller on hold, ask their permission: 'Do you mind if I put you on hold whilst I reach for the file?'
- Holding? Go back every 30 seconds, see if the caller wants to hang on or call back.
- If the caller asks if someone is there, don't ask for the caller's name and then say no! It looks like the caller is being avoided.
- Transfer calls only when necessary and always explain why.
- Don't put your hand over the mouth piece of the phone: most times the caller can still hear – learn how to use the hold button.
- Don't eat, chew or drink whilst on the phone.
- Use professional responses: no *'byeee'* at the end of the call.
- Try and sound interested and like it is the only call you've had this week.
- Leave the office, make for the nearest call box and ring yourself up. See what it's like to call your practice. If the phone rings for more than five rings and isn't picked up, you've got a problem to sort out when you go back.

What about the workers?

It is not just patients who might have cause to complain. What about the staff? Staff may have cause to complain about badly lit car parks, the loo that keeps getting blocked, or the fact that they might have to walk down the corridor with a kettle full of boiling water to make a cup of tea. Or the rudeness of the senior partner! Plenty of scope for risk scenarios there!

More seriously, if you really want to know what's going on, ask the folk on the shop floor. The problem is, many of the 'shop floor workers' never feel able to be frank without putting themselves or their jobs at risk. Expressing concerns about the clinical performance and practice of colleagues is, now, a well known topic in the NHS. However, there are plenty of other issues that staff might have a genuine opinion or grievance about. And you need to know.

Exercise

Devise a system for collecting staff opinion and complaints. Should the process anonymise the information. If so, how? Describe how you would evaluate what they say and consider ways of feeding back.

Think outside the box and the practice

Where else do you provide services? Don't forget the places that provide services on your behalf and all the other areas associated with your practice.

Exercise

✔ Here are some of the places your practice might provide services. Do an audit of your services and add to the list.

1 Satellite clinics

2 GP birthing centres

3 GP provided community services

4 Private clinics, e.g. supermarkets

5 Prisons, armed forces

6

7

8

9

10

Consider what you might need to do to bring these places into a RM system.

Finger on the trigger

How are you doing so far? Beginning to get the idea? RM is everybody's business, involves everything you do and is about the four principles. What four principles? Look on the wall! What, not ripped the page out yet? OK, just once more:

The Four Principles of Risk Management

1　Identify the risk – *figure out what's likely to foul up.*

2　Analyse the risk – *think about what the chances are of it going wrong, its impact and does it matter.*

3　Control the risk – *is there anything you can do about it?*

4　Cost the risk – *what's the cost of getting it right versus the cost of getting it wrong?*

Yes, it's getting smaller – I'm running out of pages!

Thinking about principle number one: *figure out what's likely to foul up.* What other things, events and occurrences are likely to trigger risks for your practice? We've learned, already, that some of the risks are obvious. The folks on the shop floor will know. The clinical risks are pretty evident. Are there any more?

How can we find out? How about some brainstorming sessions with the staff?

Brainstorming – what's that?

I'm sure you know. But knowing isn't doing. A lot of groups try to use brainstorming techniques but they get it wrong. Here's the right way to do it.

Brainstorming is the creative generation of ideas relating to a single topic. Such as: 'What are the risks to children at the surgery?'

You need a facilitator (that could be you or someone who has a bit of experience in brainstorming or who has taken part in a brainstorming session before), to encourage every member of the group to come up with ideas which might solve the problem or address the issue.

This is the important bit. The deal is: <u>all the ideas, however daft they may sound, no matter how irrelevant or silly they may seem, are written up on a flip-chart, so that everyone can see them</u>. No one comments on the ideas and nothing is rubbished or trashed.

Once all the ideas have been generated, contributors have the chance to elaborate on them and the group to evaluate their merit.

A lot of ideas will be crossed out but the betting is you'll be left with some interesting and innovative solutions – and a safer place for youngsters to visit!

Exercise

 Have a brainstorming session and generate a list of likely 'risks'.

Got a little list?

OK, so you're like Nanki-Poo in the Mikado – you've got a little list of likely risks. What are you going to do with it? Well, it's your *trigger list*. A list of stuff that could give you grief. A list of potential problems. Some of the things on the list can be taken care of straight away. Some of the things on the list might need to be monitored.

Let's deal with the simple things first – the ones that can be monitored and their progress followed through. You need a reporting system.

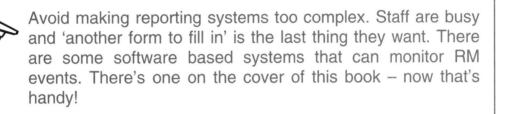

Avoid making reporting systems too complex. Staff are busy and 'another form to fill in' is the last thing they want. There are some software based systems that can monitor RM events. There's one on the cover of this book – now that's handy!

In the meantime, stick to reports that can be completed by ticking a few boxes.

Exercise

Design a reporting system. Consider who will use the system and what its purpose is. Take into account the time it takes to fill in a report. What will happen to the reports and how will action and outcomes be monitored?

A good use for the information is as a way of spotting trends. For instance, are complaints on the upswing? Do they relate to a specific person or activity?

Exercise

Devise a trend analysis system to spot trends early, to enable prompt action to be taken. How can you be sure not to over react to data, or let things go on for too long? Remember timeliness is next to Godliness – *I know your Mum told you it was cleanliness, but not in this case. Sorry Mum!*

What about the 'make you lose sleep' stuff?

Did the brainstorming throw up some things to lose sleep over? Maybe the reporting system is showing up some nasties? Consider the more serious events in the context of what to do about them. Any organisation that has not had a RM approach before can expect to be stunned at some of the things that are going on. That's the whole point of this exercise.

Exercise

 Consider a critical issue such as the unexpected death of a patient or the unplanned readmission to hospital of a seemingly well patient.

Devise a strategy to get a clear picture of what happened. Whose help would you need to enlist to produce a report? Describe your approach and what you would do with the outcome information.

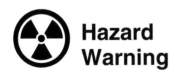 **Hazard Warning**

If you do find yourself in the unenviable position of investigating something major that may involve taking statements from staff, don't overlook how vulnerable they might feel. Consider what support networks might be needed.

What have we learned?

So, we've done our brainstorming, we've got our trigger events list and we are monitoring for trends. What next?

Learn the lessons and take action. Use the reports to implement any necessary changes. Quite often, implementing change can be a problem. People don't like change and sometimes cannot see the reasons for change.

> Remember the trigger list and the trend spotting you did in the previous exercises? You will have a lot of valuable information at your finger tips and that could be the best ally you've ever had. Show doubters the trends and their opposition should melt away. They will be able to see the reasons for action and the risks of inaction.

Wanting to change for change's sake, or because you think change might be necessary is one thing. Basing the need for change on hard evidence makes life a lot easier.

We ain't got no educashun

Some of the information you have may indicate the need for further staff training. This may impact on budgeting. Can you afford to send someone swanning off on a course? The next question is: can you afford not to? See if other practices have the same needs. Establish the position across your PCG. Can you get a group of people together and invite a guru to visit you – sharing the cost? How about joint funding one person to go and get some training, on the understanding that when they come back, bursting with new knowledge, they pass it on in some lunchtime seminars.

What about asking a pharma-co, insurance company or other supplier, to help with the cost or to do the training for you. They have armies of bright people only too keen to ingratiate themselves to you. Training is a much better deal than the usual free coffee mug or a pen!

Exercise

 Consider ways to train the organisation without it costing an arm and a leg.

Risk management checklist – eight steps to heaven

Action	Issues	Done ✔
1 Identify the hazard	• Use team brainstorming to identify potential problems • Analyse complaints data for recurring events • Talk to service users • Examine claims records	
2 Describe the hazard	Define the hazard in the context of potential risk to the: • clinician • the practice • the patient, their family carers and friends	
3 Describe existing controls	Be stripped-pine honest, if there aren't any, say so!	
4 Identify any additional measures to improve control	• What needs to be done? • What are the realistic controls? • Consider evaluating their success – how to measure them • Do you need outside help?	
5 Identify person responsible for carrying out the measures	• Who's going to do this? • Can they fit it into their 'day job'? • Do they have the skills? • What are the training implications? • What are the financial implications?	
6 Set benchmark and target dates	• Set realistic dates for improvement • Set measurable outcomes	
7 Record the findings	Keep records to reinforce progress	
8 Measure the outcome	• What have you achieved? • Is it what you wanted to achieve? • What do you need to change?	

The risk management to-do list

Action
| By when?
| Who?
| Done
|

1 All doctors, including locums, to have GMC registration verified
2 Check eligibility for all NHS lists/undertaking specific procedures such as minor surgery and child surveillance
3 Check education status (for PGEA and validity to practice)
4 All practitioners have a job description and practice agreement
5 Procedures for monitoring new practitioners
6 Check registration of staff, where appropriate
7 Ensure adequate skills for practice practitioners, nurses etc
8 All staff have job descriptions
9 All staff have copy of practice employment policies and contracts of employment
10 Staff trained in telephone manner, confidentiality, NHS issues, etc
11 Keeping up-to-date with latest guidance and clinical governance issues
12 Practice policy and procedures manual written and reviewed
13 Managing urgent/routine appointments
14 Protocol for recognising 'urgent'
15 Protocol for visit requests
16 Managing missed or cancelled appointments
17 Notifying patients of delays – policy for managing delays
18 Prescription system: for collection, noting records, review of repeat prescriptions, nurse prescribing protocols
19 Telephone advice – protocols, who can advise, noting records, call back and recall
20 Mechanism for ensuring all telephone messages are passed to the relevant healthcare professional, promptly
21 Protocol for confirming messages are received
22 Review processes to follow-up tasks delegated
23 Training in confidentiality issues
24 Procedure for labelling and sending samples
25 Patient survey and satisfaction assessment and follow-up

```
                                              Action
                                                |    By when?
                                                     |    Who?
                                                          |    Done
                                                               |
```

26 Develop team brainstorming activity to establish 'hidden issues'

27 Action

28 Develop team building initiatives to involve all staff in RM issues

29 Assign responsibility for establishing trigger issues

30 Assign responsibility for incident reporting systems

31 Establish audit for medical records

32 Establish audit for prescribing issues

33 Review complaints procedures

34 Establish 'occurrence screening' allowing for early analysis of events, prompt response to complaints

35 Review surgery based surgery procedures to include the following:

36 Demonstrating training, currency of knowledge and keeping up to date

37 Consent procedures

38 Patient information leaflets review

39 Monitor unplanned readmission and unexpected patient death

40 Patient records available when patient consults

41 Checking resuscitation and other equipment regularly and as required

42 System for checking outstanding referrals

43 Review of practice post and extraction of 'serious mail' including lab results

44 Notify patient of results

45 Ensure prompt receipt of medical record (regular FP22 check against new registrations)

46 Protocol for routine sorting of medical records

47 All record entries dated and signed

48 Managing note shortcomings in practitioners

49 Documentation of findings in medical records – positive and negative

50 Repeat medication records

51 Management of software and PC systems, site licences and millennium compliance

52 Back-up systems

53 Procedures for recognising staff deviation from practice policies

54 Staff appraisal system

55 Procedure for ensuring return of patient records

56 Procedure for managing complaint/claim staff safety out-of-hours

EIGHT STEPS FOR IMPLEMENTING A
RISK MANAGEMENT SYSTEM

1   Identify key risk areas – *use brainstorming and staff interviews, review past incidents, check claims histories, talk with patients*

2   Identify key trigger events – *look for trends, analyse national incidents for potential local impact*

3   Implement an incident reporting system – *encourage no blame culture, encourage 'near miss' reports, involve all staff*

4   Investigate high risk events – *take care in getting statements from staff, consider support networks*

5   Monitor and analyse reports for trends – *trend spotting is vital to RM solutions, be stripped-pine honest, don't fudge unpleasant truths and don't rush to judgement*

6   Implement changes in practice as necessary – *managing change is the biggest risk of all. Ensure everyone understands the reason for change*

7   Education and feedback to staff – *audit training and education needs. Folk generally don't come to work intent on fouling up. They often do it out of ignorance*

8   Involvement of outside agencies with RM expertise as necessary – *don't expect to have all the answers. Network with other practices, roll-out solutions and compare problems with others in your PCG. Use a guru, but watch the costs*

SECTION 2

This section looks at some specific issues where there is a higher than average risk of something going pear shaped and looks at ways of dealing with them

 Time for a coffee break and a flip through the pages . . .

1 If it wasn't documented, it wasn't done

Risk management and clinical documentation

We all know the jokes about doctors' handwriting. Well, times are changing and a higher standard of record keeping is becoming par for the course.

As the NHS changes, so the need for more accurate records is stressed.

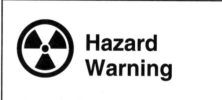

Hazard Warning

Research shows that up to 40% of medical negligence claims are rendered indefensible due to documentation problems. Make a note of that will you!

Here are just a few of the changes that can impact on record keeping:

1 The greater involvement of patients in making choices about their own care

2 More patient centred, rather than task oriented care

3 Patient access to their own records

4 The increasing use of computers

5 Clinical audit and governance

6 Commissioning healthcare within national service frameworks.

Exercise

 Take one of the above factors and consider the potential consequences of poor record keeping in that environment. What could you do to avoid the problems?

What constitutes 'records'? Well, the rules say records should contain the famous five:

1 Identify the patient
2 Support the diagnosis
3 Justify the treatment
4 Document the course and results
5 Promote the continuity of care among healthcare providers.

Clinical records do not have to show the patient made a wonderful recovery *(although speaking as an occasional patient that is always nice!)*, they just have to show that the clinician acted reasonably, according to accepted standards – regardless of the outcome.

> The Access to Health Records Act 1990, that came into force on 1st November 1991 means patients have the right to see medical records kept about them <u>since that date</u>. They already have the right to see computerised records since the Data Protection Act of 1984 came into effect. Poetic coincidence that date isn't it? Data protection, stuff about us held on computer and 1984. All very George Orwell!

By the way, records are supposed to be complete, legible and accurate. The complete and accurate bit doesn't seem to be a problem – it's the legible bit we seem to have most trouble with! *(More later!)*

What else about records? Well, here are five more things they are supposed to do:

1 Meet legal and service requirements – *more of which I will delight you with later*
2 Provide information and communication between all healthcare professionals
3 Document the care as a basis for planning care and treatment
4 Allow for the evaluation and progress of the patient
5 Change therapies where effectiveness has not been demonstrated.

Let's get risky

Now we know the rules, what are some of the potential risks that we need to manage? Here are a few ideas, to get the juices flowing:

Problem	Solution?
Identify the patient without risk of error – look out for two patients with identical or very similar names	Make sure the notes have a **name hazard** sticker on them
Ensure the continuity of care	Accurate and contemporary notes, comprehensive
Enable communication between different professional groups	Clear data on what has been prescribed and done, the responses to treatment and a demonstration as to how clinical decisions have been arrived at
Allow for concurrent or retrospective review	Chronological records of a sequence of events, the factors observed and the response to treatment
Allow for the collection of data for research/ education purposes	Clarity of all elements
Sufficient information to protect the practitioner and the patient	Allow for patients to examine their own records and be involved in their care through informed consent. Research shows that where patients have made a complaint and been shown their records, they are less likely to pursue a complaint if the records are complete and clear. Where they are scant and indecipherable the patient is more likely to become suspicious and pursue the complaint

Nothing else could go wrong with documentation, could it?

You wanna bet!

Take a look at this lot!

Legibility

It's not too much to ask, is it? Why can't docs write nicely? They say docs write badly so they can get off the hook – they write a squiggle and pretend it means anything. The trouble is, it might mean 'anything' to a fellow medic seeing the same patient and trying to work off the notes.

Some docs still think medical records belong to them. They don't, they belong to the Secretary of State for Health and the patient has a perfect right to see them and understand them and a colleague has a reasonable expectation that they will be helped and not hindered by a set of medical notes. Misinterpreting a set of notes can be disastrous. Hypertension can easily be muddled up with hypotension. See what I mean?

A great trick some barristers play is to ask a healthcare professional to read an entry they wrote, perhaps years earlier. If they can't do it, they look really stupid – and dangerous. Ouch!

Exercise

Describe how you would arrange to sample medical records for legibility. Consider issues such as patient confidentiality.

Also, how would you approach a colleague suffering from *chronic-handwriting-unreadability-itis?*

Absence of information

The job doesn't stop with the pills or treatment. Here's a good question: 'What happened?' Where a course of treatment is given or there is an expected outcome, it is important that the outcome is documented. If not it is difficult for another practitioner to determine any improvement or deterioration in the patient's condition.

If you do end up in court, swearing that your course of treatment for Mrs Bloggs was wonderful and she made a full recovery, even though she swears to his Lordship that she still can't do the shopping, it is nice if you noted the dear lady's recovery in her notes. Makes for a much stronger case and makes your lawyer a happy chappie (or chapess).

Exercise

 The advent of clinical governance arrangements and the requirements of the National Institute for Clinical Excellence, now mean that the effectiveness of treatments must be fully documented. Consider what changes in practice behaviour will be required for you to comply. How would you arrange to audit the outcomes?

Blank spaces

This is a great trick. A few well chosen spaces can be left and filled in at a later date. It used to work quite well. The problem is, these days, ink can be forensically dated. Mmmm, embarrassing if a word in the middle of the sentence can be shown to be three years younger than its parent paragraph! Do you like porridge? I think they still serve it in prison, don't they?

Alterations to the record

Never destroy, or rewrite a previous record. Tempting though it may be. In the past it might have been possible to get away with it. The problem is, these days patients have access to their records. If they turn up in court with a copy of their records that look nothing like the copy you have brought along from the practice – well, it's back to the porridge for someone!

Inappropriate abbreviations

You could fill another book with jokes about the abbreviations used by doctors to describe their patients and their conditions. In fact I think someone has. Well, joke over! If others who need to see the records, for the purposes of patient care, cannot understand them – well you can figure that one out for yourself.

For example:

PID	Pelvic Inflammatory Disease
	Prolapsed Intravertebral Disc
RTC	Return to Clinic
	Radio-therapy commenced
	Routine Terminal Care

. . . makes all the difference, doesn't it?

Lack of identification

Is this too basic to even mention? Problems will arise when the patient's name or identification number is not at the top of the page of the record or the lab result. Why do I mention it? Because the medical insurance folk tell me they are forever dealing with the fall-out from this problem.

Biased notes

Even if the patient is a complete pain in the sit-upon, try not to use phrases such as *'the patient is always complaining'* or *'the patient is too demanding'*. Yup, I know, it may be true. But it doesn't sound good when it's read out in court! Puts you in a bad light, don't you think?

Confusing the subjective with the objective

Subjective, defined as: *due to the conscious, thinking or perception of real or external things imaginary*

Objective, defined as: *external to the mind, actually existing, dealing with outward things, not thoughts or feelings*

. . . pretty classy, eh?

Put into the real world: *appears to be eating the diet*. What type of diet, quantity, supplements given?

Or, *dressings appear soiled*. Type of soil, colour, smell, volume. (*Ugh, disgusting, so pleased I'm not a Doc!*)

What about, *had a good week*. Improved by, no complaints, pain, discomfort. Analgesics effective in controlling pain.

So, now you know what not to do.

Exercise

Devise a method to audit medical records. What criteria would you use and what outcomes would you look for?

You know you've got it right when the records start to look like this:

Patient history is pertinent to the condition	Present and past medical history Family history Social consideration Relevant medication and known allergies Condition on admission
Progress notes	Changes in condition POSITIVE and NEGATIVE Details of unusual occurrences or injuries Record of insertion/removal of drains, catheters, injections
Response to care and treatment	Therapeutic and special diagnostic tests Specimens obtained, where sent, path' results, treatments given etc
Evidence of patient consent	Consent form conforms to practice policy and informed consent guidelines Pros and cons of procedure discussed and documented Consent obtained by Dr or practice nurse, with authority to carry out the procedure Correct procedure for patients under 16 years Special statutory requirements, such as detention under the Mental Health Act 1983
Facts of an injury/incident	If Mrs Brown falls entering the premises and sustains an injury and there are no witnesses, then the record must show: • Observations made • Seen by the doctor, treatment prescribed, investigations carried out and their results • Continued observations and outcome
Discharge criteria met	Fit for discharge Able to cope at home Suitable support provided, if necessary Community nurses, social services informed as appropriate
Patient/carer's teaching and understanding	Record patient/carer's understanding and giving information leaflets Include information about: • Medications • Diet • Restrictions on activity, importance of rest/exercise • Specific treatments such as colostomy care, catheter care, dressing changes
Clarity of documentation	Write legibly in black ink Write signature clearly, every time information is documented Accurate record of time and date of entry Alterations made clearly No unauthorised abbreviations No subjective statements
Discharge or treatments against medical advice	Document discussions with patient, family and carers as appropriate

Exercise: Develop this table as a matrix for medical record audit

On the dog and bone

It's the fashion. The Prime Minister likes it and the Department of Health thinks it is the latest wheeze. What Tony wants, Tony gets. He wants loadsa nurses and docs on the dog and bone *(phone to you)*, sorting out problems on the blower *(stop pretending you're a toff, you know it means the telephone)*.

Can be very risky. This needs a bit of RM if ever anything did. Are you game to try and sort out the flu from meningitis over the phone at three in the morning? Or tell the difference between the result of six pints and a Vindaloo and a heart attack?

Taking a history from a patient over the phone is not easy. The flying doctor at Wallamboola Base in Australia will tell you all about it! Dealing with requests for a home visit is full of traps too. The GP may not have previously met the patient, or the person making the call may be upset. Deciding whether or not to visit is, sometimes, a tough call. The decision is a clinical one, based on the doctor's judgement after questioning the patient or caller – plus a fair bit of intuition.

Sometimes the decision not to visit can be fatal. In such cases clear documentation as to why the decision was made may save a career.

THE RECORD SHOULD BE BASED ON THE SEVEN GOLDEN STEPS

1 Time the call was received from the patient/caller

Yup

2 Time the doctor returned the call

3 Findings following questioning, including relevant medical history and when last seen by a GP or hospital

4 Instructions including call back if there is no improvement, follow up at the surgery etc

5 Clinical reasons for not carrying out a home visit

6 If a decision is made to carry out a visit but there is likely to be a delay due to workload/prioritisation, inform the patient of the delay and document the discussion

7 If the patient says they cannot wait – alternative arrangements

Exercise

Draw up guidelines for dealing with out-of-hours calls and requests for home visits. Write them from the perspective of a new or locum member of staff wanting to work within safe and acceptable parameters for themselves, the surgery and their patients.

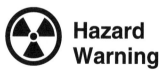 **Hazard Warning**

All NHS bodies and employees have a common law and professional duty to protect the confidentiality of the patient.

The Caldicot Review of Patient Identifiable Information recommended that NHS organisations should be held accountable through clinical governance procedures, for continuously improving confidentiality and security procedures governing the access and storage of personal information.

So you've got all those lovely records . . .

When can you get rid of them?

Do you mean you haven't read *HSC 1998/217*, what do you do all day?

OK, I'll make it easy for you, here's a summary:

Type of record	Minimum Retention Period
Maternity	25 years
Children and young people: including paediatric, vaccination & community child health service records	Until the patient's 25th birthday, or 26th if an entry was made when the young person was 17, or 10 years after the death of a patient if sooner
Treatment for mental disorders within the meaning of MH Act 1983	20 years after no further treatment considered necessary, or 10 years after the death of the patient if sooner
Records for those serving in HM Armed Forces	Not to be destroyed
Records for those serving a prison sentence	Not to be destroyed
All other personal health records	10 years after the conclusion of treatment, the patient's death or after the patient has left the country

What else? Here's a checklist:

1 Current patient records must be stored on the premises
2 Protected from fire, flood and damp
3 Records for patients no longer registered, store in line with the above requirements. All NHS records must be returned to the Health Authority within 14 days
4 Non-paper, computer records password protected and back-up files held off-site
5 Health Authority responsible for performance of any outside storage agencies.

Indefinite storage of records is a costly business and the Department of Health takes the view that this cost would far outweigh the cost of liabilities likely to be incurred in the occasional case where the defence is hampered by the absence of records – so now you know.

☢ Hazard Warning

When documents are destroyed they must be incinerated or shredded with appropriate safeguards for confidentiality throughout the procedure.

2 Cutting the risk out of surgery

Risk managing general practice surgery

Yes, I know, diagnosing measles can get boring. What better way to cheer yourself up than with a bit of carving and needlework. Just the job! The patients like it too. No long waits, nice and convenient and it keeps the docs entertained with learning something new.

But! Yup, there is a but. Sorry to be such a killjoy . . . practice surgery is a fertile ground for foul-ups and complaints. Let's look at some of the RM issues around practice surgery and start to put together a RM strategy.

What does it take to do the job well? There are seven headings:

1 Good organisation
2 Suitable equipment
3 Suitable facilities
4 Adequate support

5 Good preparation
6 Adequate surgical skills
7 Comprehensive record keeping

That's not too difficult, is it? Pity a lot of docs can't manage it all! Risk management is about the four principles: remember them? OK, don't worry about turning back, I know it's a big effort for you. Here they are again:

The Four Principles of Risk Management

1 Identify the risk – *figure out what's likely to foul up.*

2 Analyse the risk – *think about what the chances are of it going wrong, its impact and does it matter.*

3 Control the risk – *is there anything you can do about it?*

4 Cost the risk – *what's the cost of getting it right versus the cost of getting it wrong?*

. . . that's the last time!

Here are some practice surgery checklists to take you through the obvious

Do you know what you're doing?

A practitioner has to satisfy him/herself that he/she is fully competent to perform the procedures in question. So, how do you get up to speed?

- Referring to texts and photographs
- Seeking expert tuition
- Observing a consultant
- Doing cases under supervision
- Agreeing protocols with local surgeons
- Organising continuing support and access to advice

If something does go wrong a doctor can expect to be asked to demonstrate how *'competence was acquired'*. Nice phrase!

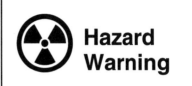 **Hazard Warning**

Any medical practitioner who carries out a surgical procedure for which they have had inadequate training, or possesses insufficient skills, is in breach of their terms of service, in breach of their duty of care and may be considered negligent.

The days of 'see one, do one, teach one' are probably numbered. Clinical governance will take care of that!

What can you do? Well, it's more a case of what you'll get paid for doing. The 1992 NHS Regulations list the following:

Incisions	Abscesses, cysts, thrombosed piles
Excisions	Cysts, lipomata, warts, ganglions, toenail removal, naevi, papillomata, dermatofibromata & similar lesions, plus skin lesions for biopsy
Aspirations	Joints, cysts, bursae, hydrocoeles
Injections	Intra-articular, peri-articular, varicose veins, haemorrhoids
Curettage, Cautery & Cryotherapy	Warts, verrucae and other skin lesions such as molluscum contagiosum
Other procedures	Removal of foreign bodies, nasal cautery

And . . . other procedures that the Health Authority thinks that you are competent to do and represents better value for money than carting a patient off to hospital. But it must be with their agreement.

Where you gonna do all this stuff?

Here's a facilities checklist:
- Room of adequate size – *no regulations here but 14 m² is generally considered reasonable*   *Yup* ✓
- Well-lit
- Affording privacy
- Operating theatre table/couch
- Operating lights
- Dressing trolleys
- Instrument cupboard
- Work surfaces
- Storage cupboards
- Sharps bin
- General waste bin
- Washing and hand drying facilities
- Disposal of sharps and dressings in an approved manner
- Recovery facility for patient who may feel unwell after the procedure

Plus, an assistant! Essential to:
- Hold instruments
- Assist with sutures or ligatures
- Adjust lighting
- Prepare instruments and dressing packs
- Ensure specimens are labelled and packed for dispatch

Equipment:
- Appropriate to the task
- Serviceable
- No rust
- Meets appropriate British Standard
- Clean and fully sterilised (*if not disposable*), preferably autoclaved or hot air ovened
- Sterilisation equipment regularly maintained – *records to prove it is*

- Or instruments and packs sterilised using a local Central Sterile Supplies Department
- Equipment requiring regular checking – *inspected to an agreed timetable and the results recorded*
- Resuscitation equipment regularly checked – *records etc*
- A resuscitation sheet displayed on the wall for all staff to see
- Room to perform resuscitation

Assessment, information and consent

OK

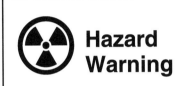

Hazard Warning

In the case of vasectomy a written consent must be obtained covering the following points:

- The operation should be regarded as permanent

- Not be regarded as successful until 2 negative sperm counts have been obtained, results in writing

- Alternative contraception should be used in the meantime

- Risk of late reversal if the tubes spontaneously rejoin

Where possible have the consent signed by the patient and the partner. If partner declines, record the reason why.

- Is the lesion suitable for surgery in the practice, or better done in hospital?
- Particular circumstances making it unwise – excessive scarring or risk of malignancy?
- Does patient have unsuitable medical history – compromised circulation, complex medication?
- Undertake examination in advance of the procedure
- Full explanation to the patient about what is to happen
- Advice to patient on after effects, journey home, time off work, timing of suture removal
- After the procedure, record it in 'Operator's Book', however minor. Record: date, nature of the procedure, type of anaesthetic used, name of operator and assistant, note of complications

- Details of the procedure fully recorded in the patient's notes
- Patient leaflet explaining post-operative care and effects such as pain or bleeding
- Patient's consent secured and recorded
- Children over 16 may sign their own consent but if they are under 18 it may be wiser to discuss surgical procedures with parents, with their consent

Anaesthesia

Modern anaesthesia has revolutionised surgical practice and made all this fun stuff in the surgery possible. The most popular is lignocaine, used either plain or with adrenaline and either infiltrated into the field of operation or used to block a particular nerve.

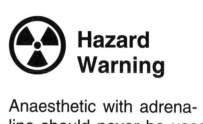

Hazard Warning

Anaesthetic with adrenaline should never be used for digital, nasal, ear tip or penile anaesthesia. These structures are at risk from tissue necrosis because they are supplied by end arteries.

The maximum safe dose of lignocaine for a 70 kg adult is 200 mg (equivalent to 20 ml of 1% lignocaine). If adrenaline is included in the anaesthetic the maximum dose increases to 500 mg (equivalent to 50 ml of 1% lignocaine).

Local anaesthetic may be supplemented by intravenous diazepam to produce an analgesic effect. The patient remains conscious but has no recollection of the procedure afterwards. Diazepam may cause hallucinations, including those of a sexual nature – so the operator should be accompanied during the procedure.

What about general anaesthetic? Best advice is forget it. Today it is generally thought inappropriate outside hospital.

Technique

Here's a checklist:

OK

- Where appropriate mark lesion with an indelible marker
- Follow natural skin creases or Langer's lines, avoid nerves and arteries in superficial locations
- Scrub up and clean operation site with antiseptic
- Ensure incisions are elliptical to prevent 'dog ears' during closure
- Consider 'cosmetic' outcomes
- Suture carefully with appropriate material and ensure they are not left in-situ for longer than necessary

Histo-pathology

Many surgical procedures undertaken at the practice will involve the removal of a skin lesion. It is the surgeon's responsibility to do the following:

Done

- Ensure the sample is placed in a suitable transport medium (supplied by the lab)

- Correct labelling of the specimen

- Ensure the result is received

- Act on the result if further treatment or referral is required

- Record the transfer of the specimen in the operation book

- Notify the patient of the result (not obligatory, but good practice)

What happens when it all goes wrong?

Back to Murphy's Law. If it can go wrong, it will! If the doc follows accepted guidelines, has adequate training and technique and has properly managed the environment and the procedure, there's isn't too much to worry about from the RM point of view. However, if a complication does arise, here are the golden rules:

- Inform the patient of the complication without embellishment

- Apologise for the unforeseen event

- Fully record and examine the complication or damage before deciding whether to attempt a repair or refer it to a specialist colleague

- Ensure the complication is treated and rectified as soon as possible.

3 Come on over to my place

Cutting out the risks associated with home visiting

Home visits – to go or not to go, that is the question.

From anything up to a quarter of complaints about GPs involve a punch up over a request for a home visit, or the events surrounding one. Requests for a home visit from a patient who is 'a bit off colour', is up and about and has three cars in the drive and four adult, sober relatives in the house are inclined to get up any doc's nose!

Some docs enjoy home visits – they see it as part of a medical tradition, it gets them out and about and is a relatively relaxing part of their work.

When is a home visit appropriate? What do the rules say?

Doctors' Terms of Service specify:

. . . services rendered by a doctor may be provided at his practice premises or, *if the condition of the patient so requires*, at the place where the patient was residing when he was accepted by the doctor or any other place where he has agreed to visit.

No one seems very sure what the bottom line is. Try this.

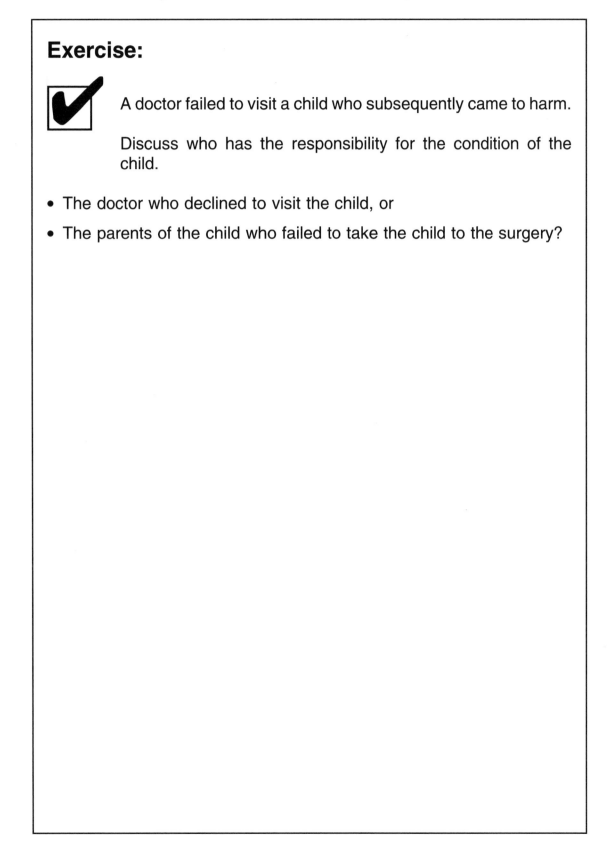

Exercise:

A doctor failed to visit a child who subsequently came to harm.

Discuss who has the responsibility for the condition of the child.

- The doctor who declined to visit the child, or
- The parents of the child who failed to take the child to the surgery?

Here are six tips aimed at RManaging out of hours and home visit calls:

---

1 Develop a set of practice criteria, agreed by partners or the out of hours co-operative

2 If a home visit is refused, document the reasons clearly

3 If sought at night, ask yourself whether the patient would have received a visit rather than a surgery appointment, had the request occurred during the day

4 If a parent does not bring a child to surgery after a visit request and then calls a second time, it is often the sign of a serious problem

5 It is better to argue with a patient after an unnecessary visit than to have to defend yourself when a necessary visit was not carried out

6 **If in doubt, go!**

---

4 Who said you could do that?

Risk management and consent in general practice

GPs undertake millions of procedures every week. Some will involve little more than a cursory glance, others may require a detailed examination. Obtaining a specific consent from the patient, to be touched or treated, in every case is not a practical proposition. Consent can be expressed or implied. Implied consent may be assumed when a patient uncovers some part of their body, without the prompting of the doctor, to allow an examination to take place.

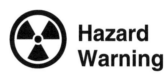

Hazard Warning

It would be easy for a patient to give a consent to a treatment without properly understanding what the consequences might be. In that case, consent without a full explanation is unlikely to cut much ice in court.

Expressed consent may be sought where an intrusive examination is to take place and where an untoward consequence or adverse outcome is a risk.

When consent is sought it should include the following elements:

OK

- A clear explanation of what is proposed

- An explanation accompanied by drawings, photographs and in a language the patient can understand

- If the patient's first language is not English and the doctor cannot speak the patient's language, engage the services of an interpreter, perhaps a relative, where appropriate

- Invite the patient to bring a relative or friend

- The person making the explanation need not, necessarily, be the person who will carry out the procedure – but they must have a comprehensive understanding of what is proposed

- Written consent is not essential but it forms a useful part of the consent process. Giving the patient a form to take home may help them to consider the implications of what is proposed

- The information must be sufficient for the patient to be adequately informed

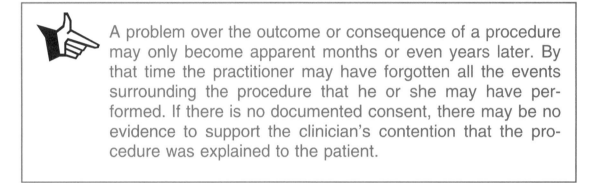

A problem over the outcome or consequence of a procedure may only become apparent months or even years later. By that time the practitioner may have forgotten all the events surrounding the procedure that he or she may have performed. If there is no documented consent, there may be no evidence to support the clinician's contention that the procedure was explained to the patient.

How much to say?

How much should a practitioner tell a patient? No one wants to frighten a patient, but they are entitled to know the facts and the doc may put him/herself at risk if he/she does not disclose sufficient information. The answer is not simple.

There are three key things to remember:

- Tell the patient what a reasonably competent practitioner would have told the patient in a similar position

- Always answer a direct question

- It is acceptable to omit a reference to a risk of treatment if the doctor considers that it would be harmful to the patient's health to do so.

What does the law say? Basically, consent is based on *self-determination* and a *respect for individual integrity*. There are three separate elements:

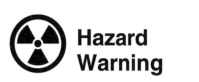

Hazard Warning

A competent adult may refuse any treatment offered to them, however certain the clinician might be that the treatment is necessary – it cannot be imposed on them. Even if the treatment is necessary to preserve life or health, the adult retains the right to refuse.

- A willingness to undergo treatment

- An understanding of the nature of the treatment

- Sufficient information to make an informed consent.

That's the routine stuff out of the way. What about the more difficult cases? An incompetent adult may not make decisions for him/herself.

In order to decide if an adult is incompetent, there are two factors to take into account.

- The first is their understanding of what the procedure is and why it is being recommended

- and the second, their appreciation of the consequences, outcomes, adverse effects and risks.

The important thing to remember is that the care of an incompetent adult cannot be delegated to another adult.

It is for the doctor to decide and to act in the best interest of the patient. This may involve the doctor consulting, widely, with family, carers and friends of the adult.

. . . and trying to make an assessment of the factors that the patient would have taken into account if they had been in a position to do so.

It gets trickier . . .

For a child under 16 years, the courts have given guidance in the shape of the 'Gillick' case. The basics are:

- The rights of self-determination for the child are recognised

- The parents' rights can be overridden

- Children under 16 may have sufficient maturity to understand the matter requiring a decision

- They may have sufficient intelligence and awareness to understand the consequences in order to give consent

- The self-determination of a child is confined to consent in law although it may be reasonable and proper to respect a child's refusal to undergo a particular procedure.

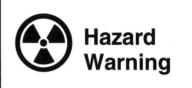 **Hazard Warning**

Under 16 and wants the pill?

If a girl under 16 does not want her parents to know of her request for contraception the doc should respect her wishes. However, they should make every effort to encourage parental involvement and make sure the girl understands the consequence of her actions. The doctor does not require a written consent to provide contraception. The doctor is advised to keep a very good record and notes based on a careful assessment.

The important thing is: keep a crystal clear set of records of any conversations of this type of issue. If parental wishes conflict with what is regarded as 'reasonable clinical practice' – the doctor must act in the best interest of the child.

Some religious groups have strong feelings about some medical procedures, such as blood transfusions.

Provided the doctor can demonstrate that they have considered all the issues, including alternative treatments and taken everyone's view into account – the doctor must act in the best interest of the child.

End of story!

Prescribing and medication errors

One of the sweet mysteries of life!

Seriously, no one seems to know how bad (or good) the risks are on prescribing and medication errors. Pharmacists will tell you, anecdotally, that they regularly save a GP's bacon by pointing out errors on scripts – who knows what the truth is? No one collects data centrally. There is a definition of medication errors:

A preventable prescribing, dispensing or drug administration error

. . . there, I bet you feel better for knowing that!

However, as the incidence of error is dependant on the definition and no body collects all the data – we ain't got a clue! Guess what? There is some US data – well there would be wouldn't there! Goodness knows how good it is, but here it is anyway:

Incidence of medication errors (US):

- Prescribing .3%–2.5% of all items prescribed
- Dispensing 1%–12% of items dispensed
- Administration 12.5%–25% of items administered.

Seems like someone should put a bomb under the administrators! Anyway, we can identify some of the major causes of risks in prescribing:

- Quality of handwriting
- Similar drug names
- Verbal orders
- Using non-approved abbreviations
- Poor prescription charts
- Prescribing in unfamiliar disease areas
- Poor clinical pharmacy services.

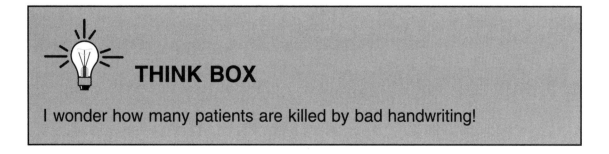

THINK BOX

I wonder how many patients are killed by bad handwriting!

5 Fancy a day off?

Risk management and locums

A day off or an evening out? Why not? Go and introduce yourself to those strange people you live with, they are called your family! They are quite nice people really! Once you get to know them!

How about a hobby?

- Bungee-jumping
- body piercing
- knitting
- weight-lifting parties
- gardening
- restoring vintage cars
- basket work
- wine making
- Morris dancing
- train spotting
- marathon running . . .

There's loadsa stuff outside the surgery, in the real world. It just takes time.

That's the problem – time. Who minds the shop whilst you are way?

And, it's not just things like parachute jumping that might be occupying your time, there is the little matter of who runs the PCG and how you play your part in this great new venture. Primary care management looks like it could be heading for free-fall, unless people like you get out of the surgery and do your bit.

That means you can't be in two places at once.

💡 THINK BOX

Department of Health guidance tells us: a PCG can be run by a chairperson in two days a week. *(Ho, Ho!)* That means for eight days a month the chair-doctor will be engaged in the life saving pursuit of sitting in meetings and shuffling paper. Indeed, for 96 days a year the chair will be debating, instead of diagnosing. Assuming there are something like 480 PCGs in England, I make that 46,080 days that will be given over to paper and given up by patients.

If a GP takes on the role of one of the six 'other' PCG Board members, the guidance indicates that each can expect to be engaged on PCG business two days a month, or 24 days a year. For a total of 480 PCGs this means about 69,120 patient contact days could be lost. The doctor will be away, working at that part of the cutting edge of medicine which involves a table, a cup of tea, a ginger biscuit and a biro.

Let's assume, in a busy surgery the average GP sees something like 25 patients in the morning session and 25 patients in the evening surgery; about 50 patients a day are likely to turn up to see their doctor. However, if, between them, chairs and PCG members are absent for a total of 115,200 days a year, locked in battle with serious medical activities like rationing, disciplining so-called profligate medical colleagues who do not comply with PCG rules about allocating practice funds, the impact on patients will be huge.

Half a million patients a month – equal to the whole population of Sheffield, or about six million patients a year, very nearly the population of London – will not be seen by their regular doctor, because their regular doctor will be regulating the spending of the petty cash.

Six million patients will be seen by an informed stranger, called a locum.

Ah, the locum!

What are the risks associated with a locum and what do we do about them?

First, give some thought to the fact that the locum is likely to see a patient when they are at their most vulnerable. How they behave, on your behalf, is certain to have a bearing on how the patient perceives your practice. One brush with a rude or abrupt locum condemns the whole practice. Sorry, but it's true. Back to the American management guru Tom Peters. He says '*perception is everything*', and he's right.

Locum checklist

Get this right and you'll go some of the way to being able to take the day off for your aerobics class, tattoo lessons or PCG play away days, with a clear conscience.

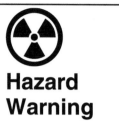

Hazard Warning

One brush with a rude or abrupt locum condemns the whole practice. Sorry, but it's true. Back to the American management guru Tom Peters. He says '*perception is everything*', and he's right.

Now, wouldn't that be nice? No, I don't mean a PCG play away day, I mean a clear conscience.

☢ Hazard Warning

Here's some stuff you need to know about locums. The data relates to locums in NHS Trusts, not primary care. It comes from an Audit Commission report. Unfortunately, there is not much data around on the quality and other factors of locum services in primary care, but if this is anything to go by it should sound a note of warning, caution, concern (call it what you like) in primary care.

- On a typical day in the NHS 3,500 doctors will be working as locums in England and Wales
- The annual cost is £200m (*I figure this translates into about £1 in £12 spent on staffing costs in Trusts going towards the cost of locums*)
- About 70% of long term locums between the ages of 35–55 had qualified overseas
- The single greatest factor why overseas doctors became locums was because they couldn't find a permanent job
- Among UK qualified locums, the greatest factor was to be able to combine work and domestic agenda.

The audit commission concluded:

Whilst there was no evidence that the care from a locum was of a lower standard of care from permanent staff, it did recommend a tightening up of the appointment and supervision of locums together with enforcing arrangements for performance review.

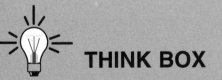

THINK BOX

If we were a bit better at *'family friendly'* policies, would we see as many UK staff working as locums? Would it be better for them to be employed permanently? What would that mean for your practice?

Locum and out of hours services

25 fings to fink about

Check it out

1 Are planned absences from surgery agreed as part of the practice policies?
2 How are locums selected? How is the process audited?
3 Are locums retired friends who like to come in for a few odd days to 'keep their hand-in'?
4 How can you be sure their practise is safe and up-to-date?
5 If locum agencies are used, how were they selected?
6 What are the criteria?
7 Was there competition in the selection process?
8 Are locums appointed on the basis of recommendations from an agency?
9 If so what is their criteria?
10 Does the practice play a part in the selection process?
11 Who plays that role, what is their experience?
12 Who is responsible for ensuring the locum's GMC registration is verified?
13 How is the locum's experience and knowledge verified?
14 What is done to check on the performance of the locum?
15 Is the patient's perspective taken into account – how?
16 Is the locum's performance against practice norms compared?
17 Is the locum more likely to admit patients to hospital?
18 Does the locum prescribe more drugs?
19 What procedures are in place to evaluate trends in the performance of the locum?
20 Are out of hours services provided on a co-op or agency basis? What is the reason for the choice?
21 What are the out of hours protocols?
22 What are the reporting mechanisms?
23 Who monitors the budget and costs?
24 Can you claim cash from the out of hours development fund?
25 What do patients think of your out of hours services?

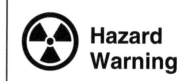 **Hazard Warning**

The GP practice principal is ultimately responsible for the performance of the locum.

In a co-op the principal responsible for the service carries the can.

6 It's not what you know

Actually, these days, it is!

Risk management and continuing professional development

Clinical practice is changing all the time. New drugs, new therapies, new diagnostics, new software, new everything. Keeping up to date was never easy and it isn't getting any easier.

Trouble is, you're going to have to! The Gods of Whitehall have a new bit of guru-speak for you: *continuing professional development* or CPD.

CPD is a cornerstone of clinical governance (the lazy person's guide to the mysteries of CG is on page 131).

Make a coffee and have a look – prepare to be horrified!

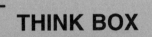 **THINK BOX**

Continuing Professional Development, or CPD as it is called, is something of a mystery. Docs get points for going to meetings, many sponsored by pharma-cos, that turn out to be really not much more than a bit of a jolly. Can you partner a pharma-co to do something really useful around CPD and CG. Most of the pharma-cos are gagging to get on board the PCG train and many of them have a genuine desire to get a better understanding of CG. Are there ethical reasons that prevent a closer working relationship with a pharma-co, or is a well defined and sensible relationship something to work for? Does your practice have a policy about such matters? If not, why not?

. . . see what I mean? Spooky, eh? All that business of statutory duty of quality and the other good stuff about making sure every one is up to speed. If you, or one of yours, fouls up and it can be established that you hadn't taken reasonable steps to keep up to date with best practice – the best thing to do will be to try and get a job on a Tuna fishing boat in Japan.

What can you do? Well, here is a list of folk that will probably be able to lend you a hand, point you in the right direction and give you some ideas. Now is the time to go and be nice to lots of new people – oh, what fun!

- Regional Education and Development Groups
- Education and Training Consortia
- Post Graduate Deans
- Local Medical Workforce Advisory Groups

And, don't forget the director of Human Resources at the local Trust hospital.

They will know a thing or two about all this – and it's about time we gave them something useful to do!

But, don't tell 'em I said so!

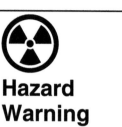

Hazard Warning

If you, or one of yours, fouls up and it can be established that you hadn't taken reasonable steps to keep up to date with best practice – the best thing to do will be to try and get a job on a Tuna fishing boat in Japan.

There is another group of folk to whom you can turn for some help – go and see them. More meetings!

- Clinical Tutors
- Royal College Tutors
- Regional Directors of Education and Training

Exercise

The NHS has a whole network of library services that can be used to support CPD.

Devise and carry out an audit of library services and design a programme to develop linkages with the various reference and library resources to make the pool of knowledge accessible and available.

Consider the role of IT in this process.

 Time for a cup of coffee and to read the NHS Human Resource Strategy Document: *The New NHS – working together, securing a quality workforce for the NHS*. Who thinks up these titles?

Heaven help us (or them). Stuck for a copy, try the HR department of a Trust or download a copy from the Department of Health website.

What, not wired? No access to the Internet. Consider early retirement.

Exercise

 Set in the context of CPD, what are the training and education needs of the practice? Devise a method of matching the organisational requirements around CPD and the skills needed, by the staff, to deliver the agenda. Tough job? Yes it is. But there is no point trying to deliver an organisational agenda without knowing whether, or not, the troops are up to it. So, tough exercise yes but a tougher world without it.

 You can have a second coffee, or something stronger, whilst you figure this one out!

Exercise

Each employee should have a training and development plan. How would you assess the training needs of an individual? Do they have to be job related, or can the development be 'personal development'?

Exercise

What benchmarks can you establish and put in place to ensure the individual is benefiting from development training?

How are you going to do all this?

Here are four good questions:

1 Who is going to do all this?
2 Should you develop a lead person to take on the responsibility?
3 Does it have to be done by someone within the practice, or could it be done by contracting out?
4 Is it really a role that is better done on a pan-PCG basis?

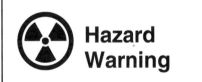

Hazard Warning

Being out of date carries a serious risk and is increasingly difficult to defend in a court of law.

7 We ain't got a barrel o' money

Risk management and money

Level 1 PCGs have only an advisory role in helping the health authority to do the job. PCGs that take on a devolved responsibility for 40% or more of the PCG unified budget will be regarded as big boys and girls at level 2.

There's a catch! To remain at level 2 the PCG will have to expand the responsibility for the devolved budget to 60% in the following year.

This is starting to get interesting! And a bit risky. Let's look at how to manage the money risks.

The NHS works in a cash limited environment, nothing new there. But PCGs now have the opportunity, challenge, worry, call it what you like, to manage the budget and cope with the little trials and tribulations of life such as: emerging high cost treatments for a small number of patients, unpredictable fluctuations in demand, movements in prescribing costs, new technology, emergency events, pay and price increases, litigation and an unhelpful press stoking up demand for this or that. Welcome to the real world!

Not all of the risks can be met or managed by PCGs or health authorities. Some of them are risks that Trusts and other providers will carry. The important thing is to make sure everyone knows, in advance, who does what. Figuring out who carries the can for what is called a Financial Risk Management strategy. Here's what you do:

- Assess the likely level of risk
- Decide where the risk is best managed
- Create risk reserves and devise procedures for monitoring budgets through the year and when to release the reserves
- Agree how any calls on risk reserves will effect the following year's budgets.

Exercise

 Make a list of potential financial risks and indicate where you think the risk should be managed.

Exercise

 Potentially, there are two ways to manage financial risk. Either the health authority can create a pool to cover the risks of all the PCGs in their area. Or, they could devolve the responsibility to the PCGs and let them create their own reserves.

List the advantages and disadvantages of the two approaches.

Exercise

- On what basis would you calculate the size of the contribution from each PCG to the pool?

- How would you clarify which budgets and services are covered by the reserve?

- Define under what circumstances you would allow access to the reserve.

- Develop some criteria for access.

- How would you monitor the arrangements?

- If the reserves were not called on, how would you manage the un-spent balances?

Good risk financial management is about two things. A sensible appraisal at the start of the year and a grip on budget management throughout the year.

Year on year PCGs are expected to balance their books.

End of story. . .

Under spending is as much of a crime as over spending but where, during the course of the year, genuine savings have been made, the good news is you get to keep them.

Ten steps to avoid being scumbered

Under what is called 'incentive arrangements', there are ten principles:

1 Reward PCGs who have taken on responsibility and done it in a clinically and cost effective manner
2 Rewards are made at the level at which the decisions are made
3 Reward value for money high quality care
4 Fits in with national and other initiatives and rewards improvements in access and equity
5 Is balanced between PCG overall and practice based improvement
6 Simple to operate
7 Be motivational
8 Reward good practices even if the PCG is poor
9 Allow for year on year performance
10 Incentivise good performers to help poor performers.

Further incentives include a prescribing incentive scheme – to keep costs down.

In practical terms what does it all mean?

If a practice gets lucky and benefits from windfall savings, all bets are off and the money goes to the PCG for redistribution. However, if they are clever boys and girls and they create savings through being good at what they do, they get to keep the first £10,000. After that it all gets a bit complex and will, no doubt, become a new battle ground for the negotiators. In simple terms, the next £70,000 of practice savings is split 50/50 with the practice and the PCG. Savings over £80,000 are up for discussion.

A couple of important points. The PCG's first duty is to spend its share of savings on bailing out over-spenders, and a practice cannot (without the agreement of the health authority), accumulate its share of the savings to save up for some mega, gold plated idea.

So you've got your savings, what can you spend the money on? Take the whole of the practice to the pub for a good night out? A week in Bermuda for the chairman and his wife? Sorry, no!

Here's the list:

- Material or equipment for treating patients: such as defibrillators, nebulisers and bits of kit and the associated consumables like that
- Lifestyle counsellors for providing advice on how to give up smoking, or get thin, or come off the booze
- Kit for the practice such as air-conditioning, vending machines and anything that makes the place more comfortable or convenient for patients and staff
- Computers and software
- Non-recurring staff costs
- Anything to improve prescribing
- Health education kit, such as tellies, videos, leaflets and the like
- Investments in premises, consistent with the Primary Care Investment Plan.

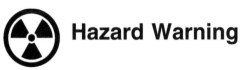

THINK BOX

If this all sounds a bit like fundholding – it was you wot said it, not me!

☢ Hazard Warning

Here's what you can't spend your ill-gotten gains on: services or kit not connected with healthcare, employment costs of existing staff, purchasing land or premises, pay-off loans or mortgages, drugs, medicines or appliances, hospital services, anything not in line with the Primary Care Investment Plan.

8 Send three and four pence, I'm going to a dance

Risk management and communications

Four-pence, what's four-pence? Old money! Old money and an old story – but true.

Apparently, during one of the campaigns in the First World War, a beleaguered group of luckless soldiers were dug in, with the enemy crawling all over them. The commander saw his only way to survive was to advance – but he needed more troops to do it. So, he sent a messenger, hot foot, with the message: 'Send reinforcements, I'm going to advance'.

The messenger had a hell of a time getting to HQ and passed the message back on a message relay arrangement, by word of mouth, from messenger to messenger.

When the message finally arrived at Brigade HQ, it said: 'Send three and four-pence, I'm going to a dance.' History does not record what happened to the troops, dug in at the front line.

Communications – a dangerous game!

Communications are at the heart of a successful consultation. Get the communications right and nine times out of ten you'll get the diagnosis right. Get the communications right and nine times out of ten the patient will go home, reassured, knowing what they are supposed to do and knowing what to expect. Poor communications are at the heart of most medical negligence claims against doctors.

Here are a few ideas to improve communications in the surgery, have a cup of coffee and a ponder

- Don't rush to judgement. Delay making a hypothesis for a couple of minutes. Be prepared to challenge your own conclusions and be willing to abandon them if they are not right.
- Ask yourself the questions the patient asks you: why now, why me, what happened?
- Let the patient make the running: allow them to voice their concerns. Often the real reason for their visit to the surgery is only revealed just as they are leaving – *'Oh, by the way doctor, just while I'm here'.*
- Listen with genuine interest – put the pen down and look at the patient – it works wonders!
- What's the patient thinking? Look for the clues.
    - ◇ Do they make eye contact?
    - ◇ Do they look anxious, sad, angry, what is their breathing telling you?
    - ◇ What about their facial expression, gestures?
    - ◇ Can you tell anything from the way in which they are dressed? Is the patient usually smart and businesslike, do they look scruffy?
- Avoid doc speak and jargon.
- The patient, like a customer, is always right, so let them go first. Use open questions to get them started: 'Tell me what it's like when . . . ' or 'What's worrying you?'
- Listen and repeat back what they have said – this lets the patient correct anything that you've got wrong or they haven't explained very well.
- Shut up. Yes, for once in your life, button it. People often find pauses and silences difficult. If you remain silent the patient will often fill the gap with something more, or useful, or with greater clarity – or the truth!
- Try and put the patient in the driving seat and involve them in the decision making. This does not mean that you give up control of the patient's care but it does mean giving choices and helping informed decisions and that means greater patient understanding and compliance with treatment protocols.
- Remember a doc has a special place in the community. In the minds of many patients they are powerful figures, particularly for the elderly. Use the power with care. Don't sit behind a desk and surround yourself with medical kit, books and blurb from the pharma-cos.

Walk into your consulting room with a fresh pair of eyes –
does it look like a medical bring and buy sale, a teenager's
bedroom, or jumble sale? If you've had something on your
desk for more than three days – burn it. If you've got stuff piled
up on the floor – burn it. If you've got notices on a board older
than one month, burn the notice board. Never worry about
shredding memos from the health authority or circulars from
the Department of Health. If it was important they'll have kept
a copy!

- Make it easy for the patient to do what you want: think about their life style, intelligence and resources.

- Think about our American friend Tom Peters' phrase: *perception is everything.*

- Look for *'non-verbal leakage'*: this is guru speak. This guru is a guy called Peter Tate, who coined the phrase in his excellent book *The Doctor's Communication Handbook* (Radcliffe). He uses the phrase to describe the difference between what the patient says and what their non-verbal behaviour is telling you. *'No, I'm not depressed'*, whilst sitting, shoulders slumped, a sad fixed expression – exuding gloom. That's what Tate is telling us about.

- What do your words mean to the patient? *'Won't'* means *'might'*, *'can't'* means *'could'* and *'shouldn't'* means *'probably will'*!

- You cannot share the patient's beliefs unless you know what they are.

- Be prepared to say, *'I don't know, but we'll find out'.*

- Note the use of the plural noun 'we'. Use 'us', 'together', 'we'.

- What are the practice leaflets like? Seriously, are they grubby little photocopies? Pharma-cos are a great source of leaflets and the long term and chronic disease societies have loadsa stuff.

> ⚛ ## Hazard Warning
>
> Oh, and whilst you are being a real saint and doing all the listening and looking stuff, don't forget to make notes both clinical and patient centred – clearly. Don't bury your head in notes in front of the patient and if you're using a computer, tilt the screen so that the patient can see it. Think about the last time you checked into a hotel and how infuriating it was when the receptionist said 'Hello, welcome, what's your name' and then buried his/her head in the computer monitor, tapping away like a demented woodpecker for what seemed like ages!

Before we leave communication – what about internal communications with staff and everybody else?

The fastest way to lose staff is to let them feel undervalued and forgotten. Don't risk losing staff because of poor internal communications.

Here's some fings ta fink about. . .

- Does the PCG Board or practice understand that there is more to communications than sending out a monthly newsletter?
- Will you develop a communications strategy?
- What will it include?
- Who will design and prepare it?
- Who will you involve in the process?
- Will you use outside consultants or experts?
- What type of mapping exercise will you undertake?
- Do you know what you want to say?
- What techniques will you use to say it?
- What are the likely barriers to success?
- What is the role of the Chair and CE of the PCG?
- Who will ensure implementation?
- What training is needed?
- What will it cost?
- What are the key outcomes?
- When and how will you review it?

AND

Do not use communications to be manipulative. Open and honest communication will allow all parties to move forward. Whether the news is good or bad, tell it like it is as fast as you can. Move like greased lightning.

Gossip rips through an organisation like a bush fire. The best way to stop it is to get there first.

By the way, PCGs have to hold their meetings in public and allow for public participation – how ya gonna do that?

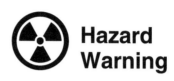 **Hazard Warning**

Understand how gossip works. In a large organisation the average employee will interact with 15 people in a day. That 15 will talk to another 15 and another 15 and so on. By the end of the week, the world knows there are going to be redundancies.

Here's some ideas

Let's be honest, very few practices have any real experience of involving the public in the development of services.

The key question is: why are we involving the public? Is it because you have to or because you see some benefit in doing it?

It is very easy to play the game and follow the rules. It is also very easy to be patronising. Involving the public means just that, involving them. This is not something the NHS, the medical profession nor the Department of Health has been good at. 'Doctor knows best' is not a phrase that will continue to have much currency in the New NHS. The truth is, the doctor often does know best but now the doctor has a mission to explain, and that means involving patients and the public. Patients and the public seldom make unreasonable demands – if they know the facts. Talk to them.

Exercise

This is a short exercise for two or more participants.

Ask them to write down five plusses about involving the public and five minuses. Collate the answers on a flip chart. Do different professionals have different perspectives about the value of public consultation? Use the headlines as a focus for brainstorming solutions about public participation and drawing some value from it.

The evidence is, the public does not rush to health authority meetings in droves. Unless you plan to close a hospital – then stand back or you will be trampled in the rush or hit on the head with a banner! Health public meetings are usually attended by staff side organisations, patients with special needs and user groups.

Here are some important Key Principles to think about

- See the community as having a potential for solving problems and not creating them. A higher level of public understanding and awareness can only make decisions more likely to be acceptable.

- The PCG's job is to enable community participation – not to control or own it.

- Try to involve the community, not just listen.

- If the community is going to feel it is making a worthwhile contribution, it must be able to set the agenda.

- You can change community perception by involving evidence from elsewhere, epidemiology and the results of trials. You may need to reshape technical evidence into a more easily understood format. But remember, the public aren't daft, so don't patronise them.

- The process doesn't come cheap. Think about crèche facilities, interpreters, management time, costs of advertising and publications.

- Take care that minority interests are not swamped.

- PCGs themselves are in an early stage of formation and will have more questions than answers. Make it clear you are seeking views and listening in order to shape your own views.

- Community well being is derived from a variety of sources. PCGs are supposed to provide the focus for agencies to work together. Make sure they are represented at communication meetings.

- Why should members of the public be bothered to attend – unless they see concrete outcomes of their involvement? Make sure they have some early signs that it is worth the trouble to be involved.

- The odd meeting here and there is not going to help. To do this properly, real involvement and communication may involve full time staff making the links, networking and developing trust and understanding.

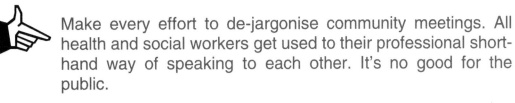 Make every effort to de-jargonise community meetings. All health and social workers get used to their professional short-hand way of speaking to each other. It's no good for the public.

- Think of involving the public as their fundamental right – after all, they are paying for the services you provide.

Still stuck for ideas on how to involve the public. Here are some thoughts:

Suggestion boxes – in shops, supermarkets, libraries – anywhere people go! Be prepared for some rude answers!

Road show and media events – expensive to produce and need a professional touch.

Open meetings of the Health Authority and PCG – the public are entitled to attend meetings but the evidence is they seldom do. CHCs send a representative and sometimes staff-side organisations turn up.

Postal questionnaires and surveys – one of the most unsatisfactory ways of gathering opinion. The technique excludes a very high proportion of the community who have poor reading skills (more than you'd ever imagine!), the young (who seem not to bother), the elderly (who have trouble reading and replying), and those whose first language is not English. Forget this one.

Health Panels – a trendy idea used by some trendy health authorities. The idea is to, randomly, select some households to serve on a panel. They are regularly surveyed and asked for their views on whatever topics interest the health authority. The panellists are not given any briefing material and the views are not much better informed than opinions that might be aired at the Dog and Duck.

Focus groups – a development of the health panel. Loved by the Labour Party and much used in industry. The group is selected (this is the bit that requires the care) and in depth dialogue techniques used to uncover real attitudes. This really is a job for the professional and is not a cheap solution. Generally the technique is used to gather views on an existing agenda rather than to uncover new needs. Marginalised groups are difficult to engage in the process.

Practice patient participation groups – selection of participants is the key. The vocal middle classes seem to dominate. Generally they address low key agenda items such as appointment systems, transport and the like.

Citizen's Juries – this is a very sexy approach. Very new New! A dozen or so members of the public are brought together for three or four days. They are selected using market research techniques, so a professional company is required to do this bit. The jurors hear from 'expert witnesses', who provide information about a specific topic. The jury then comes to a decision that is taken up by the Health Authority. This is a very high profile approach that, because it is new, attracts media attention. They are not without costs. The whole process can come to £30,000. On the down side, they involve few people and health authorities are not bound by the decisions.

Rapid Appraisal – this is a research based approach. Researchers interview and gather information from so-called 'key informants'. They could be health and social workers, shop keepers, community representatives and so on. This is an exclusive approach and depends on the line taken by the researcher.

Community representatives on committees – the CHC or some other organisation can nominate a community rep to be on a committee. Generally they bring a narrow perspective and can be overwhelmed by a large committee, used to speaking jargon. Community reps need careful induction and training. They are usually single issue members and may find it difficult to see the big picture. Remember, their first loyalty will be to the organisation they come from.

OK, so what works best?

As you can see all these approaches have their upsides and their downsides. They are either too narrow, too introspective or too costly. So what's the answer? In the best of worlds a community development approach, involving the community from the start, letting them decide on priorities for themselves, is the best. If they are in at the start they can follow up on issues and 'grow' with the solutions and the problems. They require careful thought about structures and mechanisms to make them work. However, the green field nature of the opportunities presented by PCGs would seem an ideal time to try this approach.

For a real insight into how to make all this work try ten minutes on the phone with Philip Crowley. He's at a health resource centre in Newcastle and knows his stuff! Tel: 0191 2724244, or for those who are in the 21st century:
philip@wehrc.demon.co.uk

Exercise

Devise a programme for community consultation around two contracting areas, such as teenage sexual health and services for dementia. What are the similarities in approach and how will they differ?

Does this mean a multi-faceted approach for every service area, or are there themes common to all circumstances?

PCG members may be unused to making decisions in public, or indeed speaking in public. Meetings in public can be like working in a fish tank or appearing on a stage. For most of us, neither is a natural environment.

From the practical point of view there are considerations about access and meeting times, distribution of minutes and relationships with the press and public that do require careful thought.

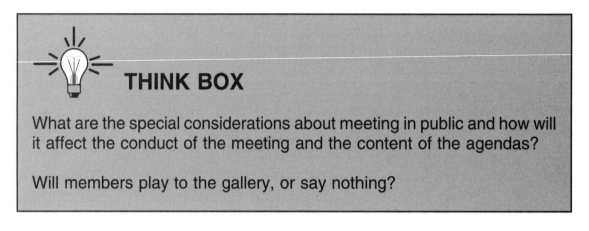

THINK BOX

What are the special considerations about meeting in public and how will it affect the conduct of the meeting and the content of the agendas?

Will members play to the gallery, or say nothing?

Come on – let's do this right!

When you think about it, health is pretty important to us all. One way or another, the NHS and associated services will play a part in our lives and the lives and well-being of our families and friends.

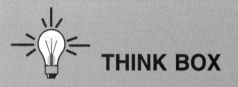

THINK BOX

How decisions are made and the consequences of them could be vital to us. BUT, and it is a very BIG BUT, none of us get a chance to vote for the people who make the decisions about our healthcare. Every five years we get the chance to chuck one lot out of Westminster and let another lot in. In between times decisions about rationing healthcare, the configuration of services and who gets what and where are left to an un-elected group of managers who do the best they can with what they've got. Can't be right, can it?

Unless we want to dig up the democratic process and plant something new (*Good idea for the next book Roy – Ed*), we've got to try and make the present system a bit more accountable. The best we can do is to open up the process so that, at the very least, we can let the public watch the decisions being made. They may not agree, but they can't say they haven't had the chance to see how decisions are arrived at.

Want to impress somebody with your knowledge? Try this

New legislation (The Public Bodies (Admission to Meetings) (National Health Service Trusts) Order 1997: No 2763 came into effect on 6th February 1998), means NHS Trusts and PCGs must have their meetings in public.

Here's how it all works

- First this is not a cosmetic exercise, open board meetings must mean the public should be able to observe the decision making process.

- It is not enough to make it just a spectator sport, the public must be able to understand the internal arguments, tensions and restrictions which lead to a decision.

- So, no fixing up the decisions in advance.

☢ Hazard Warning

Notice of any meeting of a PCG, open to the public, must be given at least three days in advance. The time and place of the meeting must be published so that newspapers are able to report the meeting's decisions. You must provide them with the agenda and appropriate papers. Under normal deadlines they will need a week's notice of meetings.

So, you've got to do it. How to do it well is the question

Here are some tips for making public meetings work:

- Make the public feel welcome. Make sure the venue is someplace easy for them to get to and the seats are comfortable and everyone can see and hear what is going on. Good public transport and easy parking. Give someone the specific task of welcoming the public, pointing out where the loos are, directing them to where they can sit. Who's a good *meeter* and *greeter* in your PCG?

- If you are chairing the meeting make some encouraging introductory remarks. If there are a lot of people there, because there is a controversial item on the agenda, say something like:

'Thank you all for coming. I know there will be some issues that are of great concern to many of you, as they are to us. I'm pleased to see so many of you have bothered to come and see how difficult it can sometimes be to make finely balanced difficult decisions and I'm pleased you will be able to witness the fact we'll do our best to listen to the facts and make a decision on our best judgement. Unfortunately we do not have the wisdom of Solomon, but we do try and use our common sense. Some of you will be pleased with what we decide, others, perhaps not. We can only try and do our best for you all.'

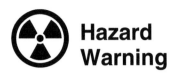

Hazard Warning

The tone of introductory remarks can set the tone for the whole meeting.

Think in advance about what you want to say.

Say it and mean it. Preparation is the key – don't try and do it off the cuff.

- If it is a routine meeting and a man and his dog have turned up, make them feel special too:

'Thank you so much for turning out. We admire your dedication! I hope, by the time of the next meeting you will have been able to persuade a neighbour, relative or friend that it is worth their time to come with you'. And give the dog a biscuit!

- Introduce the members of the board and explain their speciality. *'Dr So and So, from the Down Town Practice, Mary Smith from Social Services, Mrs Bloggs the health authority nominee'* – and so on. It helps the public understand where the members are coming from.

- Provide nameplates for board members to remind the public who the members are.

- Give the public copies of the agenda and papers being discussed.

- Consider holding a press briefing before the meeting to be sure the media understand the issues to be discussed.

- Make sure the seating is arranged in such a way that the public can follow the discussion. For example, this could mean seating the board in a horseshoe arrangement facing out towards the public and press.

- If slides or overheads are used, make sure the public can see the screen.

- Can you provide an audio loop? They can be hired for the meeting. You should do it, particularly if elderly people are likely to attend.

- What's disabled access like – token ramps or the real thing? Don't get caught out on this one. Ask a local disabled representation group to give you advice.

- Can you provide a crèche facility?

- Are there language issues? Think about translations of the printed word and perhaps translation of issues of particular interest and concern to an ethnic group.

- Have the staff been told about the meeting. Make them feel welcome too.

- What about switching the venue to make it easier for people to get to? Rotate the venues.

- If specific items for discussion are likely to be of interest to specific groups, consider holding the meeting at an appropriate venue. Young people issues in a school. Mums and toddlers, try the local supermarket. The elderly, how about a day centre? Meetings can move, you know. It's just your brains we want, not your address!

OK, so you've got them there, now what?

Unless decisions are seen to be made openly, there is no point having meetings in public. The whole idea is to let people see how it's all done and feel part of the process and to encourage public participation.

- Policy options and ideas should be brought before the Board for genuine debate and decision without rehearsal or prior agreement on the outcome.

- Arguments for and against proposals should be aired in public.

- Make the CHC your ally, involve them too.

Timing of meetings is important

Consider the possibility of some meetings being held outside normal working hours to make it easier for the general public to attend.

When can you close the doors?

This is technical stuff, so pay attention! The Public Bodies (Admission to Meetings) 1960 Act includes provision for the discussion of confidential business in private sessions.

Under the terms of the Act, a Board may resolve to exclude the public from a meeting (whether during the whole or part of the proceedings) whenever publicity would be prejudicial to the public interest by reason of the confidential nature of the business to be transacted, or for other special reasons stated in the resolution.

So now you know!

The resolution should be taken in public, and minuted. It should state in broad terms (which do not breach the confidentiality of the subject matter) the nature of the business to be discussed.

Within the terms of the legislation, members of the public and press do not have a right to speak at meetings.

However, there is nothing to stop the chair inviting contributions and questions.

Your Board may wish to make time in the agenda, at the beginning or end of meetings, when questions can be taken.

Or what about asking the public to submit written questions for you to answer?

⚠️ **Hazard Warning**

Don't abuse the powers or you will bring the wrath of the Secretary of State down upon you! Nasty!

Limit closed sessions to:

Where real harm to individuals may result. This might include discussion about particular members of staff for disciplinary or other reasons, or relate to independent reviews on complaints.

What about sub-committees?

Smart question!

The provisions of the Act do not relate to sub-committees of the main board unless all board members are members of the sub-committee. It is recognised that the subject matter of audit and remuneration committees, as well as committees looking at issues such as complaints and appointments, will in any event generally be of a confidential nature.

However, no cheating – the establishment of sub-committees should not be used as a means of diverting business which is properly a matter for the full board or to avoid issues being addressed in public. Furthermore, none of this precludes an invitation to the public to attend meetings of any sub-committee.

Primary Care Groups, which have devolved decision making powers on commissioning, are a special type of Health Authority sub-committee and the public should have access to your meetings. The law will be tweaked to sort out this anomaly. In the mean time you should behave like the big boys do and meet in public.

Anyway, you'll get used to it so that if and when you are at level 3 +, it'll come as second nature.

If you get it wrong?

Complaints from the public about access to board meetings or the provision of information about them or their proceedings should be dealt with in the same way as complaints under the Code of Openness in the NHS. That means, complaints should be made in the first instance to the senior officer, accountable to the Chief Executive, who has responsibility for the Code.

Dissatisfied complainants should take their complaints directly to the Chief Executive of the NHS body involved, who will provide them with information about how to take their complaint further to the Health Service Ombudsman if they remain dissatisfied.

The press and the media?

PCGs are new and will be taking on more of the role of the health authority. In consequence, expect an increase in Press interest.

Be like the Boy Scouts, be prepared!

Appointing a press officer who is able to foster trust with the media is a good start. At the risk of engaging the wrath of every doctor in the UK and every politically correct soul on this earth, I'm going to give you three pieces of advice. Here goes:

- Toffee-nosed docs in bow ties cut no ice with the public – especially on the telly

- Women make more convincing spokespersons than men

- It is rare that the chairman of any outfit is the best spokesperson.

Please don't send me hate mail! Successful communication is about empathy. Camelot, the Essex Police, umpteen public companies, the water utilities group and a host of others have recognised that women news readers and women teachers score higher in surveys about empathy, public trust and clarity of message than men.

Chairs of organisations might be very important in their environment but the public see them in the context of being a public servant and there is a huge difference.

As for bow ties? The image is all wrong. Docs wear bow ties to avoid ordinary ties dangling in wet bits when they are looking after you – makes good sense to me. The most unhygienic thing in the world is probably a GP's tie! But you can't look humble in a bow tie!

Exercise

Effective communications which involve positive and regular communication with the local community and all interested organisations, in particular with the media and the press, will make running the PCG a great deal less painful. The appointment of the right person is a crucial decision and will require careful thought. It does not have to be the lead person but their relationship with the leader is very important.

- Create the job description for the spokesperson.

Exercise

Planning to deal with the press and media?

The health service is always somewhere near the top of the news agenda. Whilst running a PCG may not make the national news (unless something goes badly wrong!) it is almost certainly likely to interest the local news media. The local press can be great allies – or they can make a bad enemy.

• Design a media relations policy (don't forget to add something about evaluation!).

9 Getting wired

Risk management and information technology and information systems

If the NHS were Jurassic Park its graveyard wouldn't be full of the carcasses of prehistoric monsters, it would be full of the bodies of IT procurement foul ups. The NHS seems to make a speciality of getting IT wrong. Why do you think that is?

Here are a few reasons. In the early days of IT there wasn't much IT know how in the NHS. The boys in the smart suits, working for the IT companies, saw the NHS as a soft target, flogged the systems, dumped the boxes and ran. The next problem the NHS had was it didn't really know what it wanted so it couldn't buy it. So, in guru speak, its *procurement* was all up the pole (to put it politely). Then came the 1990 NHS reforms, giving Trusts a wide range of operational freedoms, including IT procurement. Those Trusts that

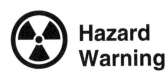

Hazard Warning

The most important IT priority is to make sure that all current systems are millennium proof.

If you don't know what I'm talking about – get back down the hole with Swampy!

If GPs buy kit that is not Y2K compliant they won't get reimbursed.

were brave enough, bought all manner of IT solutions. Each Trust had a different approach. As a consequence, the NHS ended up like an electronic Tower of Babble. Money problems and skills shortages in IT have all added to the difficulties.

The greatest enemy of IT procurement and establishing Information Systems has been the enthusiast. Usually a bored GP who 'could do IT' and was bored with diagnosing bronchitis, would position himself as the Sultan of Information Systems – heaven help us. No one knew enough to tell them to shut up and we now have thousands of systems, invented by some bloke in an anorak, working out of a shed, that won't speak to each other and fall over if you put the system under pressure.

What do we do to avoid all this?

It looks like the NHS is, at last, getting to grips with IT. The recently published IT strategy document makes it clear, IT is going to play a big part in the NHS of the future – not before time I hear you say!

A lot of the IT vendors lost patience with the NHS and a good few went down the tubes, so buying decent kit and systems ain't easy!

Already many senior managers and medics in Trusts have access to the NHS Intranet. Many GPs are already on line and the plan is that everyone will be connected by 2000. The truth is it is unlikely that it will take as long as 2000 – except in cases where GPs do not want to be on-line!

 If you work with one of those, give them a quiet dose of something nasty in their morning coffee.

PCGs will be seen as something of a Klondyke for the IT industry and no doubt an array of products will come onto the market – helping you to run your practice or PCG from the comfort of your desk, sofa, bed or beach and computer screen. The NHS has always managed to make a mess of IT procurement and another disaster is, probably, just around the corner.

PCGs have been advised not to rush into investing in IT systems until more is known of their working practices. However, there is a balance to be struck. Experience has shown that IT is better installed at foundation level in an organisation rather than added at a later stage.

PCGs will need access to reliable information. Practices, PCGs, health authorities and Trusts all share the same interest in sharing data and you need to work together to assess what they have access to already and what additional information they are likely to need.

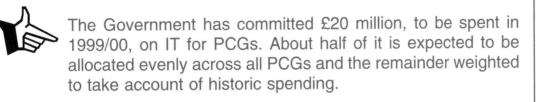

The Government has committed £20 million, to be spent in 1999/00, on IT for PCGs. About half of it is expected to be allocated evenly across all PCGs and the remainder weighted to take account of historic spending.

A proper evaluation of the practice's or PCG's likely needs is a good first step. Take account of the fact that the component practices are likely to be in differing states of *IT-ness*. Some will be developed and others not.

Keep an eye on the future to allow for expansion of systems to take into account growth and changes. Something to ask the prospective new chief executive, *'What do you know about IT'*? Beware of dabblers!

There is a specific DoH requirement that existing data systems are to be preserved. Stop collecting data at your peril.

Exercise

 Assessing the organisation's IT status

Good information technology systems are essential to a new organisation, helping it to perform efficiently and in an informed way. The best time to install them is in the start up period of the organisation's life; that way they become part of the infrastructure. The management of information by the use of technology has not been the NHS's strongest suit. However, IT will prove vital in keeping costs down and helping everyone to understand what is going on. Developments in what is available are likely to exceed the PCG's ability to pay for them but electronic patient records, tele-medicine and pharmacy management systems are just a small part of what is on the horizon.

- What practical steps need to be taken to ensure that all local practices have the necessary technology and training to be on-line by 2000?

Exercise

- How can you be certain the millennium bug will not frustrate your plans?

Some Do's and Don'ts

- Do make sure that what you already have is Y2K compliant. If you don't know what Y2K means – try a career as a lamp-lighter or wick trimmer.

- Do think hard before you buy new kit. Don't forget about the procurement problems that the NHS has already got itself into. Where can you go to for advice? Can you trust the people who are selling you the stuff? Probably not – they want to sell it, don't they? Really good independent advice on IT is hard to come by. Beware! You have been warned.

It's often not the technical specification of the software that lets you down, it is the hardware's operational memory – called RAM. Always go for the highest level of RAM you can afford and the most amount of conventional memory. Working systems eat memory, you'll be surprised how quickly it gets gobbled up.

- Do make sure you know what you want. Yes, I know it sounds banal to say it but look at it this way. Do you really need to buy the latest Pentium XYZ, with bells and whistles, or can you get a better deal by buying something with a less sexy specification? What do you really want the system to do?

- Do make sure you *futureproof* the system. That means make sure it does not have redundancy built into it. Make sure it is upgrade-able, flexible and will see you into the future.

- Do find out about the Data Protection Act – too big a subject to deal with here, call them on 01625 545745. It's one of those annoying automated switchboard thingamajigs, but stick with it and you can get a very good leaflet, or the reward for being really determined is to get to speak to a human being.

- Keeping records on computer? Do something to ensure confidentiality. Don't leave screens full of data unattended, don't give your password to the practice receptionist, or secretary, or anybody . . . (*I know you do!*) Who has access to patient records? If the price was right, who could have access to patient records? Think I'm joking? How do you think private detectives get hold of the information they do? The answer is: easy money and sloppy people.

- Do make sure you back up your files. Don't worry, too much, about backing up system files – you can always reload the system. Do make sure you back up your data. There are all kinds of automated back up systems that will do it for you regularly.

- The best advice is:
  - ◇ back up data EVERYDAY
  - ◇ critical stuff TWICE A DAY
  - ◇ and ONE DAY you'll be pleased you took this advice!

- Don't make it easy to nick your kit. Do make sure you mark it all. The local police, crime prevention Copper will be pleased to pay you a visit and help you get that sorted.

- Don't catch a virus. I don't mean one of those things that GPs say they can't do anything about. I mean real viruses that wipe out your computer. You can do something about them. First, be sure to install a virus checker. There are loadsa systems that you can install. Try looking at www.drsolomon.com. No access to the web? Go and get it, now!

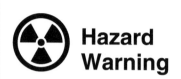 **Hazard Warning**

Do you remember the time when a TV programme got hold of the medical records of the then head-lad of the BMA, Sir Sandy Macara? I'll bet you a pint they could still do it today. What could a determined journalist with a few quid to spend and a good private detective get out of your place?

- Do fit a surge protector for your PCs. What's a surge protector? Well PCs can be sensitive to the amount of electricity going through them. The UK 'leckie system works between 220 volts and 240 volts. Although the PC reduces the voltage to something much smaller, it can be sensitive to a surge (or spike) in the supply. Nasty spikes mean blank screens and misery. PC shops and DIY stores sell extension sockets that have surge protectors and smooth out 'Spike'. Only a few quid and well worth the investment. You can also get a smart socket that stores up just enough juice for you to shut your system down with dignity and style, if the electricity supply fails. The price of a large G&T with ice and a slice – well spent.

- Don't allow games on your PCs. They can encourage the 'computer nervous' to have fun and get to grips with the machine. I guess there is an argument for that. But, they take up space and are best taken off. However, don't under any circumstances allow anyone to load their own games. For two reasons, the first is why should they be playing games in your time and second who knows what nasty viruses they might deposit on your hard disk?

What about E-mail?

If you agree that the NHS is very good at getting itself into a mess over IT, computers and technology, believe me, you ain't seen nothin' yet! There is another disaster waiting just around the corner. The millennium bug is a flea bite by comparison. The message is: it is the messages that will cause the problem.

Patient appointments, pathology results, internal messaging, ordering and countless other tasks are set to become electronic. All GPs will be hooked up with E-mail, as will most managers and hospital consultants.

Litigation, writs and battles are just an E-mail away. The problems will start internally and then the outside world will come crashing down on the heads of unsuspecting NHS management.

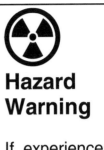

Hazard Warning

If experiences in the private sector are anything to go by, the NHS has no idea what it is letting itself in for with E-mail.

The potential for problems identified itself, in the US, last March. It was reported that the merchant bankers Morgan Stanley, Dean Witter & Co., agreed an out of court settlement with two of its employees. Reason? Some other staff had circulated a bad taste joke about African-Americans on the internal E-mail system. The aggrieved staff reached for their lawyers and the company reached for its cheque book. The court was about to decide that employers are responsible for all internal E-mail traffic, regardless of its origination. Morgan's, apparently, settled. This is just part of what the NHS can expect. Other lawsuits alleging everything from sexual discrimination to breach of confidence have been sparked by companies without proper E-mail policies and planning.

Industry has been caught unprepared by the impact of E-mail. A Gallup Poll, conducted in the US, last May, found that the typical office worker in a decent sized corporation would deal with up to 60 incoming and outgoing E-mails in a day. There are about 156,000 administrative and estates staff in the NHS (to say nothing of the doctors and nurses). That could mean, when they all get the hang of E-mail, there is a potential for nine million messages to whizz around the system, every day. Controlling the content of all of the messages is an impossible job.

Should a PCG, Trust, GP or any other health employer become involved in a court case or an industrial tribunal, electronic mail is ready to provide some more shocks. A legal device, known as 'discovery', can be used to force litigants to reveal every file, note and piece of paper they have that might be pertinent to the case in question. Nothing may be hidden. Courts can prize open your filing cabinets and archives. They can plug into your hard disk too. If the records they want to see include E-mail messages that have been deliberately erased or modified – you might find yourself in contempt of court.

Industry is spending millions setting up record management systems, policies and organisational structures to manage the invisible tide of E-mail.

The simple answer? Treat electronic messages like paper messages and file them – the gurus call it *E-archiving*. Unfortunately, this is not so simple. Deciding what to keep and what to dump becomes a major problem. What to retain, and how long for, is a policy decision the Practice Principal or PCG boss may have to answer for, in court or at the Public Accounts Committee. *(Time to buy a smart new suit!)*

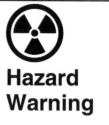

Hazard Warning

Planting a blank E-mail into a file history, makes it possible, at a later stage, to go back and fill it in with any message you like. A trick likely to fool everyone, even an experienced observer.

E-mails can easily be faked or fiddled with and printed out messages can be similarly counterfeited. A storage system that is tamper-proof does not come cheap and will eat up a storage disk faster than an American termite can chomp its way through a house.

So called E-shredding software exists and is one way of zapping messages that could come back to haunt you. However, hidden 'history' and cache files in Windows and other systems can leave a trail of clues that the determined, computer literate can follow. Emptying the 're-cycle bin' does not mean gone for good.

E-mail will become fundamental to the way the NHS runs its affairs. The service needs some rules and guidance – fast.

Here are six ideas to avoid E-fail with E-mail:

Check

1 Warn all staff, with an 'on-screen' message about the practice's rules for E-mail.

2 Make it clear that E-mail is not confidential and will be routinely monitored. More importantly, hammer home the fact that E-mail is not a substitute for the kind of conversation that used to take place in the canteen, lavatory or lift.

3 Stamp out digital gossip: bar the transmission of personal mail, jokes, smutty material and non-business messages. American experience shows staff who are offended can sue their employer – someone is bound to try a case here, sooner or later.

4 Set up in house E-training to help staff understand the rules. This might persuade a court that you have taken your responsibilities seriously. Incorporate E-mail policies into contracts of employment.

5 Install one of the new programmes to monitor E-mail for key words and phrases, to flag up offensive material.

6 Decide on archive policies now. What to keep, how long to keep it, how to keep it and who is responsible. Cost electronic archive processes and budget for it – the outlay is more than you think. Disk and tape space doesn't come cheap. But not as expensive as a few days at the High Court!

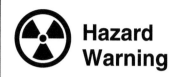
Hazard
Warning

Never, never, never, never, never, never, never, never, never, never, never, never, never, open an attachment to an E-mail that has the suffix .EXE. Unless it came from your Mother and even then be suspicious. These types of files are a favourite vehicle for the lunatic who spreads viruses.

Come to think about it don't open any attachment to an E-message if you have no idea who the sender is. These days the lunatics can infect your machine with word processing files and all manner of other stuff.

10 Hands on

Risk management and examining the patient

Seems simple enough, doesn't it? Got a painful bit, or a sore spot – go to the doc's, get your kit off, let them have a look. If only it was. Some docs get themselves into some very painful spots with this.

The first issue is that any examination has to be appropriate. Many of the claims and complaints handled (*now there's a great choice of word to use in this section – Ed*) by medical protection outfits revolve around the appropriateness of the examination.

Here are some key questions:

- Does the patient need to be 'seen' or is advice over the telephone safe and appropriate?

- Does the patient need to be examined?

- Consider the scope of the examination in the light of possible diagnoses. (*Even I know a breast examination is generally unnecessary for verrucas – Ed!!*)

- Explain to the patient your provisional diagnosis and the reason for the examination – especially intimate areas.

- Always ask permission to examine – don't assume consent.

- Medical protection insurance companies will tell you the problem is nearly always with men examining women.

The other risks are obvious, with children and sometimes gay patients.

Where is the examination to be carried out?

House vs surgery

The surgery is a more professional place to carry out an examination – it has better facilities, better light and there are people around to help, if necessary.

However, if an examination during a home visit is unavoidable (and it often will be), establish who else is in the house. If it is possible and appropriate, have them nearby. Make sure you make a note that a domiciliary examination has been carried out.

If the patient makes any untoward comment or advance, make certain they are noted in the record. Advise the patient that such comments or advances are unwarranted and unwanted.

> If the patient is persistent leave and return either with a nurse or send a partner of a gender unlikely to be part of the problem.

Chaperone?

A chaperone can be very valuable in avoiding unnecessary risks, particularly during gynaecological or breast examinations. Take care with the chaperone – there can be problems. Ensure the patient is not inhibited from telling the truth about a situation.

For example: abdominal pain in a teenager who may think she is pregnant. In some circumstances Mum may not be the best choice – try a nurse. At all costs, respect the confidentiality of the patient.

Maintaining modesty

Ensure there are screens and curtains in the surgery – if they've got to be washed or sent to the cleaners, put the number two set up, please!

Use the screen to avoid the patient undressing in front of the doctor – and that way the doctor avoids a dressing down (or worse) for a charge of voyeurism!

Use a blanket to cover the parts of the body not being examined and remove only necessary clothing. The balance to be struck here is the modesty of the patient against making sure that there is good access to areas which need examining.

Warn the patient of what you are going to do with your hands or with instruments. It's best if an intimate examination doesn't come as a surprise!

Note taking

This is a pivotal part of the examination and is dealt with elsewhere in this workbook, but it is worth a recap. A good set of notes is the difference between being able to defend a claim for malpractice and not.

Record all findings

Record all findings including the negative ones, especially when symptoms suggest a specific disease. For example: in a patient with chest pain and sweating, note that it is not a heart attack because . . .

If it subsequently does prove to be a heart attack it will be easier to defend an accusation of negligence if it can be shown that, based on the signs available at the time, the diagnosis of heart pain was not substantiated.

Explanation of findings

Explain your findings in the notes of the examination and, in particular, note any areas where the patient does not agree with you. Discuss and make clear any findings which are in keeping with a particular diagnosis or not.

Note any problems with the examination.

Note any refusal of the patient to be examined.

Note any circumstance where an examination would not be appropriate.

Further management

Make a full note of the need for any repeat examinations. For example: the need for follow-up of a breast lump. Ensure the patient understands the situation. Where possible make an appointment for the follow-up examination to be carried out.

Make full notes of the treatment plan agreed with the patient, or their relatives and carers. Ensure everyone knows what has been agreed and accepts the proposal. Note any dissent in the notes and try and deal with it.

Further investigation

If there is a need to seek a consultant referral on the basis of findings of the examination ensure the patient is fully informed about further management and what they can expect.

Complaints often stem from poor communications: the patient's expectation or understanding of events is skewed by poor communication by the doctor. Remember — if they haven't heard it, you haven't said it!

ANNEX 1

The biggest risk of all

The biggest risk to an organisation is during a period of change. When things change staff get unsettled, they leave, their motivation drops and the performance of the whole organisation can go down the pan.

When that happens all kinds of other risks creep in. The team take their eye off the ball.

 Make a coffee and read through these pages. All the changes that the latest reforms of primary care have brought mean huge challenges, great opportunities – but a whole lot-a-risk.

The section is full of ideas and exercises to help you implement changes where you work, without making it hard work.

They are aimed at building a team that can face the challenge of change together and with the minimum of risk.

If you want to know more about team building in primary care: try *The PCG Team Builder*, published by Radcliffe and written by Gareth Davis, Bill Cain and, well, I'm too modest to say!

It's all change

Risk management and change

PCGs involve change to the point where it might be redefined as upheaval! It will have an impact on every part of primary care, individuals, practices and for the professionals we work with. If you are responsible for managing a change initiative – this section is for you.

The risks in not managing change well are in the loss of motivation of staff, chaotic administration and the likelihood of errors occurring in the work of staff who are preoccupied.

This section is divided into two, reflecting the stages in the successful management of a change project.

The Key Stages

1 Define the scope of the change project – *how big is it?*

2 Diagnose the present situation – *where are you now?*

3 Create a vision of the desired future – *what does the future look like?*

4 Analyse the gap and manage the transition – *what's the difference between where you are now and where you want to be?*

5 Handle resistance – *who and what is going to make it tougher than it needs to be?*

6 Stabilise the new situation – *got there, now stay there!*

1 DEFINE THE SCOPE OF THE PROJECT

Make a start by defining the scope of the change project. This seems so obvious that even experienced change masters forget to do it! By defining the scope at the outset you will minimise confusion, identify the likely consequences and prevent trouble brewing up for you later.

The purpose of the change must be identified, the scope of the project defined and the key players who may have the power to prevent the change identified and involved.

Key questions to ask are:

- Is there an organisational problem which needs to be addressed by the change project – what is it?

- Are there defined parts of the organisation that need to change in order to address this problem?

- What are the benefits to be gained by undertaking this change – where are the wins?

- What are the consequences of doing nothing?

- Is there a price to change and is it worth paying?

---

2 DIAGNOSE THE PRESENT SITUATION

You must get a clear picture of where you are starting from, the current situation in that part of the organisation undergoing the change. This process makes it easier to identify where the problems are coming from and what needs to be changed. This will help you to decide where to focus on getting commitment to the change project.

This is the flip side of: 'if it ain't broke, don't fix it'. This says: 'treat what hurts'.

There are various levels to look at. They all impact on one another and need to be looked at as interacting systems.

Level 1 – Broad Influences

- What are the broad trends in the environment that are causing the need for change?

(Think about Political, Economic, Social and Technological trends – guru speak for a PEST analysis)

Level 2 – Local 'Stakeholder' Demands

This looks at the other organisations with which your organisation is interacting.

- How healthy is our relationship with those who interact with us (e.g. secondary care, health authorities, social services, housing, voluntary sector etc.)?

- What do they expect from us and what is the likely impact if we fail to meet their needs?

Level 3 – Culture

An organisation's culture is sometimes described as 'the way things are done around here'.

A change of culture within the organisation, or within sub-sections of it, is a major, sometimes painful, but often a necessary goal.

- Are the organisation's norms at odds with the way things need to be done in the future?

Level 4 – Core Purpose

This is sometimes spelled out in a 'mission' statement.

- Does the organisation really know and understand its purpose?

- What services/functions are we currently delivering?

- What services/functions do we really need to be delivering?

Level 5 – Internal Design

- Is the organisation designed in an effective way to deliver its objectives?

Things to look at here include tasks, people, structure, rewards, information and decision making.

Level 6 – Service Delivery

This level of diagnosis focuses on change projects aimed at specific parts of an organisation, such as Directorates.

- Is the department fulfilling its planned activity levels and performance against expectations?

- Is it delivering this activity in a way that meets the needs of its 'consumers' and 'customers'?

- Are communication processes effective both within the department and with other parts of the organisation – how do you know?

- Are individuals within the department working together effectively – how do you measure it?

- Is there an overall sense of cohesiveness within the team – does it 'feel good'?

3 CREATE A VISION OF THE FUTURE YOU WANT

Buoyed up with the first flush of enthusiasm it is easy to get a change project underway. Very often they run out of steam because no one has any idea of what they are aiming for. Change masters learn the trick of painting a picture of what the future looks like. Painting the picture helps secure commitment and enthusiasm. The whole team should be part of painting the picture – what goes in it, what colour it is, what are the textures.

Here's an exercise to help you paint pictures

This is a group exercise that involves creative thinking.

1   Ask each member of the group to think about their ideal organisation or team. *Give them 4 minutes thinking time.*
2   Ask each to share their ideas with the rest of the group *Facilitator, use a flip chart, so everyone can see.*
3   Identify key similarities and differences.
4   Create a shared vision of the future.

- Write here your thoughts about the future vision for your team/ project.

---

4 ANALYSE THE GAP AND MANAGE THE TRANSITION

When you have a clear picture of the current situation and the desired future you have the starting and end point of your project. Now you are ready for the fourth stage – identifying the gap between where you are and where you are going. We move, now, into managing the transition.

To establish the specific steps, undertake this 'gap analysis'. Go back to the previous exercises and look at what you need to do to finish the journey and arrive in your picture!

OBJECTIVE REVIEW

What needs to be done?	Objectives	By whom/By when?

 Make sure someone accepts overall responsibility for ensuring that the plan is implemented.

Communication

Effective communication is critical to the success of any change management project. Remember the Hazard Warning about how fast gossip can rip through an organisation?

Here are some 'gossip beating' decisions for you to take

- What do we need to tell people? – *usually everything, because if you don't tell, someone will.*

- When are we going to tell them? – *the best advice is 'as fast as you can'.*

- Who is going to tell them? – *the best guide is 'the person with most authority', this is not a good time to hide.*

- How are we going to communicate? – *in person is always best, it's tough and takes time but pays its own reward. If not, there are always meetings, newsletters, E-mail. People worried about change like to read what's going on in the messenger's eyes, not on a piece of paper.*

5 HANDLE RESISTANCE

People resist change for all sorts of reasons. They are not very difficult to define and many of them can be anticipated. Planning to handle resistance is the change master's way of making sure resistance doesn't hold up progress.

Here are some ways to get commitment to change and reduce resistance:

- Involvement – *make people feel part of what is going on*

- Visioning – *share the vision of the future, paint the picture*

- Communication – *tell 'em what's going on, remind 'em and tell 'em again!*

- 'Treating what hurts' – *don't change for change's sake – do the bits that need doing*

- Knowing how individuals respond to change – *think about how you reacted to change, other people will feel the same way: unsure, cautious, worried, resentful, perhaps even relieved!*

- Encouraging people to develop new relationships – *take the best of the past into the future and emphasise the difference with new working partners.*

Key question to ask:

- What are the main barriers to change, how can we minimise them?

6 STABILISE THE NEW SITUATION

Finally, the project needs to be evaluated, lessons learned for future projects and the situation consolidated before embarking on any more change. Change piled upon change will cause discomfort and morale will take a dive.

Key questions to ask:

- What lessons have we learned from the project?

- What worked well and what worked less well?

- What would you like to have done differently?

- Are there any development needs for individuals now that the project is up and running?

- What have I learnt about myself during this project?

ANNEX 2

Clinical governance supplement

Here for the price of one book, is nearly two – all the top line details on clinical governance.

If you want the low down on clinical governance and to try out £500 worth of software for free, get a copy of:

Making Sense of Clinical Governance
Radcliffe Medical Press
(Tel: 01235 528820)

Written by . . . I'm too modest to say!

Making Sense of Clinical Governance

Clinical governance is a cornerstone of RM. If you haven't read the various bits of Guidance and other stuff on CG, avalanching out of Whitehall, here is the *Dummy's Guide* to Clinical Governance. Rip it out and stick it on the fridge door with one of those funny magnet things, or stick it on the notice board in the office – to make it look like you know what you're talking about:

- Processes are to be put in place to integrate quality into the organisation's processes – it's not a departmental issue any more. Now, it's everybody's business

- Quality is a lot about leadership and that leadership is to stem from clinical team level

- Evidence based practice, backed up by ideas and evaluated innovation, will be systematically cascaded through the NHS

- Clinical risk reduction programmes will be introduced

- There will be a greater openness in detecting and investigating adverse events

- Patients will be listened to and lessons learned from their experiences

- Poor clinical performance will be detected earlier, to protect clinicians and patients

- Clinical governance is the key theme in professional development

- Improvements to the quality of clinical data captured.

In short, the NHS is finding out what industry has known for years – quality is everybody's business.

OK, that's the basics – what else?

None of this is going to happen over night. There is a lot that is good in the NHS but a lot of it ain't so good. So, the idea of CG is that it is to be 'developmental'. This is the Department of Health's way of saying 'we know it's going to take time'. The Department of Health are also saying that although they know it is going to take time, that's no excuse for not doing anything.

So, there are some benchmarks on the way.

One good thing (or perhaps it is not) is that the Department of Health is not being prescriptive. In other words, they are not defining the exact methods that are to be used. They are setting out a framework along with some key principles and the rest is up to you.

THINK BOX

If the NHS is serious about CG and quality, is it right to leave so much of the implementation up to the locals? Is this how Marks and Sparks do it? How can there be consistent quality in the NHS if everyone is being left to do their own thing. On the other hand, how much store is to be set against the ownership of a quality strategy? If folk don't own it, they won't do it and mean it . . .

THINK BOX (*I said it before and I'll say it again*)

'Whistle blowing' – now there's a phrase to conjure with! Who in their right mind wants to be a whistle blower? Do you want to be branded a whistle blower? I bet you don't and neither does anyone in their right mind. We might have serious concerns about the professional performance, or capabilities, of our colleagues and we may want to bring those concerns to the attention of someone senior in the organisation. But we don't want to bear the tabloid newspaper brand 'whistle blower' – let's find another phrase.

So, in short, here are all the important bits – on one page:

Clinical governance is:

- Everyone's business
- Involves patients and service users
- Ignores departmental and service boundaries and works across them
- Involves everyone in developing their professional capabilities
- Continuous and evolving in its quest for improvement
- Finding out what works best and doing it, every time
- Based on evidence
- Transparent and open.

Clinical governance is not:

- A stick to bash the docs with
- Another management fad
- A 'blame' thing
- Tribal
- An excuse for not doing things
- Up to someone else to do
- Keeping quiet about things that go wrong.

Clinical governance recognises:

A quality service is built by: being open about the strengths and weaknesses of what we do; being determined to improve by adopting and sharing the best practice we can find; making our own contribution more valuable through continuous personal development, comparing ourselves with the best; and by listening to the people we serve.

And here is what it 'looks' like . . .

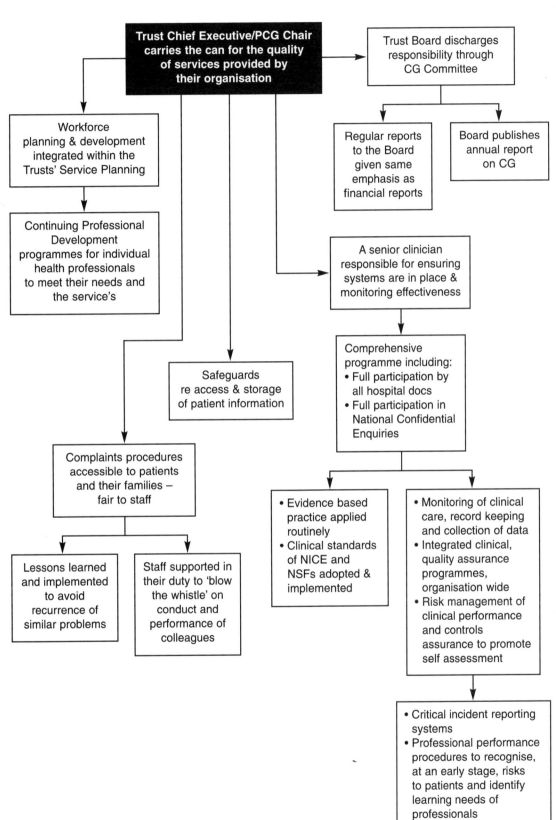

Rainy day reading or a word from Mystic Meg

Go and make a cup of coffee, come back and sit in a nice comfy chair. I want to talk to you . . . I'll wait.

 OK, do I have your undivided attention?

Over the page you are going to find a loada stuff which doesn't concern you – yet. Not yet, but I'll have a few quid on it that it will!

It's all about *controls assurance* and other grungy sounding stuff for Trusts and health authorities. At the moment, it does not concern practices or Primary Care Groups. However, when PCGs progress from the Toys-R-Us and early learning stage of PCGs at levels 1 & 2 and move into the real world of budget holding and life in the fast lane at levels 3 & 4 and PCTrusts (tomorrow the world), you don't have to be Mystic Meg to guess that it is worth an each way bet that some of this will start to apply to you too. So, best you understand it now and start putting the systems in place sooner rather than later.

Actually, on second thoughts forget the coffee, you'd be better off with a stiff gin. Anyway read on and tell me, one day, you won't have to do it . . .

Controls assurance – what the %*## is it?

Controls assurance is an all encompassing concept based on best governance practice. It is a process designed to provide evidence that NHS organisations are doing their *'reasonable best'* to manage themselves so as to meet their objectives and protect patients, staff, the public and other stakeholders against risks of all kind.

Got it?

Let's put it another way . . .

Fundamental to the process is the effective involvement of people and functions within the organisation through application of self-assessment techniques to ensure objectives are met and risks are properly controlled. Chief Executives of NHS Trusts and Health Authorities are currently required to sign, on behalf of the Board, a controls assurance statement in respect of the system of internal financial controls in their Annual Accounts. This requirement is now extended to wider risk management and organisational controls covering *inter alia* aspects of non-financial, non-clinical risk, by the production of a controls assurance statement to accompany the Annual Report from 1999/2000.

As if you didn't have enough to do . . .

The shadowy Gods of Whitehall behind all this are a group who delight in the name of the NHS Executive Controls Assurance Team. Easily mistaken for the Gestapo, they actually are a very nice group of people who realise you've already got nine million things to do. So, to make your job a bit easier they have been developing a 'control framework'.

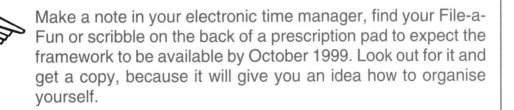

Make a note in your electronic time manager, find your File-a-Fun or scribble on the back of a prescription pad to expect the framework to be available by October 1999. Look out for it and get a copy, because it will give you an idea how to organise yourself.

Oh, by the way, another Tip:
You can get on the Web and access
open.gov.uk/doh/riskman.htm
which has a link to the main Department of Health circulars database – a very helpful place to have a root around, full of useful NHS Executive and Department of Health paraphernalia.

Incidentally, you can also get from there to an interesting site dealing with the Turnbull consultation document on risk management and control for Plcs listed on the stock exchange . . . see it's not just the NHS doing this, the world has gone RM mad.

Joined-upness

The Gods of Whitehall take the view that financial controls, quality controls and organisational controls are linked functions. Nothing new here, industry has recognised these facts since Montague Whitmore first advised manufacturers on cost accounting in 1870, Alexander Hamilton-Church taught Lancashire industrialists how to use budgets in 1898 and Harvey Preen published 'Reorganisation and Costing' in 1907 – *Ooooh, impressed, eh!*

Here's how it works. Clinical governance provides a framework within which organisations can work to improve and assure the quality of clinical services for patients. Implementing and maintaining effective risk management and organisational controls is fundamental to ensuring the success of clinical governance, providing a solid foundation upon which to build an environment where quality care can be provided and clinical excellence can flourish.

Someone seems to have realised that 'getting the organisation right' will significantly increase the likelihood of meeting the needs of patients. There – no rocket science, just common sense.

THINK BOX

The 'common thread' linking clinical governance and wider controls assurance is risk management. The Gods of Whitehall define risk management for Trusts and health authorities as *'the culture, processes and structures that are directed towards the effective management of potential opportunities and adverse effects'*. Actually I think they pinched it from the Australia/New Zealand Standard 4360:1999 Risk management. Anyway, do you have a problem with that definition? I don't see why. All of this is aimed at Trusts and health authorities – but you can see how it could easily apply to PCGs and PCTrusts, eh?

You will be used to the idea of an holistic approach to medicine. Now you have a new phrase to conjure with – *holistic risk management*.

Meaning, encompassing both 'clinical' and 'non-clinical' aspects through extending the control framework to include standards for clinical risk management, including clinical audit and clinical incidents, complaints and claims recording, investigation and analysis. Expect all this lot to fall in on your head in the early part of 2000.

OK, so what's this gonna do for ya?

Here are some of the benefits:

1   reduction in risk exposure through more effective targeting of resources to address key risk areas
2   improvements in economy, efficiency and effectiveness resulting from a reduction in the frequency and/or severity of incidents, complaints, claims, staff absence and other loss
3   demonstrable compliance with applicable laws and regulations
4   enhanced reputation through public disclosure of achievements in meeting objectives and managing risk

and perhaps

5   increased public confidence in the quality of services provided by the NHS.

Now tell me that don't feel gooooooood!

Controls assurance is designed to give Chief Executives of NHS organisations a handle on what's happening in their organisations. Don't forget they are the *accountable officers* and are the ones who can expect a funny, career limiting, half hour with the Public Accounts Committee if it all goes pear shaped. I'm sure you can see which way the wind is blowing. *(Can you 'see wind'? – Ed)*

Who's going to check all this?

Trusts and health authorities will set up internal audit groups, supported as necessary by in-house specialist expertise in fields such as estates, facilities, health and safety, risk management and infection control, and by 'external' expertise from organisations such as NHS Estates, who will be responsible for the verification of organisational controls assurance statements. PCGs can expect health authorities to encompass PCGs, at levels 1 & 2, in these arrangements.

> Expect the Audit Commission to play a role in externally reviewing the arrangements for controls assurance during 2000/2001. Ugh . . .

Regional Offices of the NHS Executive will monitor the implementation of controls assurance in NHS Trusts and health authorities. In due course, expect implementation in Primary Care Groups and Trusts, monitored by health authorities. Those nice folk at the NHS Executive Controls Assurance Team will, centrally, monitor and evaluate the overall implementation of controls assurance across the service.

The Cadbury Committee (No, not about giving boxes of chocolates to nurses) reported on the *financial* aspects of *corporate* governance in 1992. They defined corporate governance as 'the system by which companies are directed and controlled' and identified three fundamental requirements for good corporate governance in organisations:
1 internal financial controls
2 efficient and effective operations, and
3 compliance with applicable laws and regulations.

Sounds like good advice for a PCG hoping to juggle budgets and play with the taxpayer's hard earned pounds.

Subsequently, the Greenbury and Hampel Committees fiddled with the 'Cadbury Code'. And Bingo, we now have the 'Combined Code of Principles of

Good Governance' for Plcs, organisations and the like. They used a shed load of words to say:

1 'The board should maintain a sound system of internal control to safeguard shareholders' investment and the company's assets'

2 'The directors should, at least annually, conduct a review of the effectiveness of the group's system of internal control and should report to the shareholders that they have done so'

3 'The review should cover all controls, including financial, operational and compliance controls, and risk management.'

As if that wasn't enough, the Turnbull Committee has recently published a consultation document containing further guidance on these principles. The final guidance is expected by late summer 1999. Turnbull will reinforce the principle that all controls, including risk management, should be the subject of review. Reviewing the effectiveness of internal control is the responsibility of the board having regard to any information provided by the audit committee, or any other board committee. Internal audit's role is seen as evaluating the risk and monitoring the effectiveness of the system of internal control. The Turnbull report will conclude that an objective and adequately resourced internal audit function should be in a position to provide the board with much of the assurance it requires regarding the effectiveness of the system of internal control.

As this is all for Plcs you may well ask what's it got to do with the good old NHS? Well, the NHS has embraced the principles of good governance and will comply with all this stuff.

By:

1 developing a framework of corporate accountability

2 improving the organisation and staffing of internal audit, and

3 developing *controls assurance*, built on worldwide best practice relating to all internal controls (*not just finance*) including risk management.

So, now you know – time for another stiff gin?

There's a lot more to all this – keep an eye on it. It will change your life!

Here is a digest of some of the Health Service Guidance dealing with risk management

Series	Title
LAC (98)21	*The New NHS: modern, dependable* on developing primary care groups
HSG (97)6	NHS health and safety issues
HSC 1998/070	*Corporate Governance in the NHS* on controls assurance statements 1998/1999 and 1999/2000
HSC 1999/021	*Insurance in the NHS* on employer / public liability and miscellaneous risk pooling
HSC 1999/069	*The Year 2000 Problem* on testing of IT systems, estates systems and medical devices
HSC 1998/198	*Commissioning in the New NHS* on commissioning services 1999–2000
HSC 1999/074	*The Year 2000 Problem* on continuity and contingency planning for medical devices in use within the NHS
EL (97)22	*Destruction of controlled drugs*
HSC 1998/188	*The Year 2000 Problem* on management of primary engineering services
HSC 1998/092	*NHS Direct: second wave pilots invitation to tender*
HSC 1998/065	*The New NHS: modern, dependable* on establishing primary care groups
HSC 1998/030	*Guidance notes for GP commissioning groups*
FDL (97)23	Bi-annual letter of cases referred to the NHS Executive Headquarters for write off approval and summary of the analysis of frauds reported to HM Treasury by government departments 1995–96
MISC (97)35	*Corporate Governance in the NHS* on controls assurance statements [HSG(97)17]
HSG (96)12	*Directions on financial management in England*
HSC 1999/088	*Lessons to be learned from losses and fraud cases*
LAC (99)15	*Winter 1999/2000 emergency services & planning for the millennium holiday*
HSC 1999/095	*Winter 1999/2000 emergency services & planning for the millennium holiday*
HSC 1999/059	*Year 2000 Problem* on ensuring GP practices have compliant clinical systems
PL CO (97)2	Advisory Committee on Dangerous Pathogens (ACDP) guidance *Infection risks to new and expectant mothers in the workplace: a guide for employers*
EL (97)55	*Corporate Governance in the NHS* on controls assurance statements
HSC 1998/174	*Insurance in the NHS*
MISC (97)60	*Purchaser financial development group*
HSC 1998/224	*Better blood transfusion*
HSG (95)48	*Information management and technology (IM&T) procurement and private finance*
HSC 1999/028	*NHS Direct: final stage of national roll-out*
FDL (97)31	*Definition of NHS trust management costs 1998/99*
HSC 1998/021	*Better health and better health care: implementing 'The new NHS' and 'Our healthier nation'*
HSG (95)28	*Key messages for community fundholders*
EL (97)39	*NHS priorities and planning guidance 1998/99*